MW01502829

Refractive Keratotomy for Cataract Surgery and the Correction of Astigmatism

Robert M. Kershner, MD, FACS

Refractive Keratotomy for Cataract Surgery and the Correction of Astigmatism

Robert M. Kershner, MD, FACS
Orange Grove Center for Corrective Eye Surgery
Tucson, Arizona

SLACK Incorporated, 6900 Grove Road, Thorofare, NJ 08086-9447

Managing Editor: Amy E. Drummond
Publisher: John H. Bond
Project Editor: Peter T. Christy

Kershner, Robert M.
    Refractive keratotomy for cataract surgery and astigmatism/ [edited by]
    Robert M. Kershner.
        p.   cm.
    Includes bibliographical references and index.
    ISBN 1-55642-237-7
    1. Cataract--Surgery. 2. Astigmatism--Surgery. 3. Cornea--Surgery I. Kershner,
    Robert M., 1953- .
    [DNLM: 1. Cataract Extraction--methods. 2. Astigmatism--surgery.
    3. Astigmatism--prevention & control. 4. Keratotomy, Radial. WW 260 R332 1994]
RE451.R44   1994
617.7'42059--dc20
DNLM/DLC   94-15787
for Library of Congress   CIP

Printed in the United States of America

Published by: SLACK Incorporated
                6900 Grove Road
                Thorofare, NJ 08086-9447

Last digit is print number: 10   9   8   7   6   5   4   3   2   1

This book is dedicated to the first loves of my life,
my wife Jeryl, and my two daughters, Shaina Beth and Emily Rachel.

Contents

Chapter 1 1
The Physiological Basis of Refraction
Robert M. Kershner, MD, FACS

Chapter 2 13
Incisional Keratotomy Effects on Corneal Curvature
 and Refractive Power of the Eye
Spencer P. Thornton, MD, FACS

Chapter 3 25
Keratolenticuloplasty
Robert M. Kershner, MD, FACS

Chapter 4 43
Arcuate Keratotomy for the Correction of Pre-existing
 and Postcataract Astigmatism
Spencer P. Thornton, MD, FACS

Chapter 5 51
Reduction of Preoperative and Postoperative Astigmatism
 for Cataract Surgeons
R. Bruce Grene, MD
Richard L. Lindstrom, MD

Chapter 6 63
Arcuate Keratotomy—The Method, Technique
 and Instrumentation
Daniel S. Durrie, MD
D. James Schumer, MD

Contributing Authors

Daniel S. Durrie, MD
Associate Clinical Professor
University of Missouri
Hunkeler Eye Clinic
Kansas City, Missouri

Harry B. Grabow, MD
Assistant Clinical Professor
University of South Florida
Medical Director,
Sarasota Cataract Institute
Sarasota, Florida

R. Bruce Grene, MD
Assistant Clinical Professor
University of Kansas School of Medicine
Grene Cornea
Wichita, Kansas

Robert M. Kershner, MD, FACS
Associate Clinical Professor
Department of Ophthalmology
University of Utah Medical Center
Chief, Section of Ophthalmology
Northwest Hospital
Tucson, Arizona
Director,
Orange Grove Center for Corrective Eye Surgery
Tucson, Arizona

Richard L. Lindstrom, MD
Clinical Professor of Ophthalmology
University of Minnesota
Attending Surgeon, Phillips Eye Institute
and Minneapolis Veterans Medical Center
Minneapolis, Minnesota

D. James Schumer, MD
Hunkeler Eye Clinic
Kansas City, Missouri

Spencer P. Thornton, MD, FACS
Thornton Eye Surgery Center
Nashville, Tennessee

Acknowledgements

The author would like to acknowledge the contributions of my colleagues who gave up their time to help create what we feel will be one of the definitive textbooks on the correction of astigmatism with cataract surgery.

I thank my patients for their support of our efforts to make emmetropia a reality. I thank my staff for their hard work in keeping my office running smoothly through the many hours of dictating, transcribing, reviewing and editing that this project required.

Last, but not least, I wish to thank Amy E. Drummond, Managing Editor, Peter T. Christy, Project Editor, and John H. Bond, the Publisher of SLACK Incorporated for their dedication in seeing this book to completion, and their fruitful comments, suggestions and encouragement.

RMK
Tucson, Arizona
March, 1994

About the Author

Robert M. Kershner pursued his undergraduate studies at Boston University and received his Masters of Science and Doctor of Medicine degrees with honors at The University of Vermont College of Medicine. He completed his Internship in General Surgery and obtained his Specialty in Ophthalmology at The University of Arizona Health Sciences Center in Tucson. He was Chief Resident in Ophthalmology at The University of Utah Medical Center in Salt Lake City.

Dr. Kershner has authored many scientific articles on the treatment of eye diseases and is a frequent contributor to health columns. He has written several chapters in textbooks on eye surgery and is the editor of the *Video Textbook of Microsurgery*. Dr. Kershner travels internationally as a lecturer in microsurgical techniques to other ophthalmologists. He has developed several microsurgical instruments and is an innovator in single piece, capsular bag intraocular lenses.

He is certified by the American Board of Ophthalmology, the American College of Eye Surgeons, a Fellow of The American Academy of Ophthalmology, and a Fellow of The American College of Surgeons. He is an active member of The Arizona Ophthalmological Society, and American Society of Cataract and Refractive Surgery. Dr. Kershner is Chief of the Section of Ophthalmology at Northwest Hospital in Tucson, Associate Clinical Professor of Ophthalmology at the University of Utah Medical Center in Salt Lake City, and Director of the Orange Grove Center for Corrective Eye Surgery, Tucson, Arizona.

Preface

History has turned a page, as cataract surgery evolves from creating aphakia to permanently correcting pre-existing refractive error. Incremental change in surgical technique over the past decade has caused ophthalmic surgeons to rethink how we perform our surgery and control its ultimate outcome, the vision of our patients. The increased use of phacoemulsification has forced us into smaller and smaller cataract incisions. At one time, multiple suture closure of a cataract incision would inevitably result in several diopters of postoperative astigmatism. This required spectacles or contact lens correction to enable clear vision. As incisions became smaller, the amount of iatrogenic astigmatism correspondingly decreased. With single suture closure, the smallest amount of induced astigmatism finally became reality. But we did not stop there. Sutureless cataract surgery created, for the first time, an astigmatically-neutral incision. Surgeons were pleased to discover that the astigmatic refractive error following cataract surgery could equal the pre-existing refractive error. But this too would not remain the *status qou*. The cataract incision, now 3 mm or smaller, has moved onto the cornea from the limbus and away from the sclera. This clear-corneal incision gave surgeons, for the first time, the opportunity to permanently alter corneal curvature.

The hero of the decade is the greatest change in modern cataract surgery—the incision. The advent of capsulorhexis, hydrodissection, one-handed intercapsular phacoemulsification, and flexible intraocular lenses capable of implantation through incisions of 3.0 mm and smaller, have all contributed to the acceleration of cataract surgical technique into the 21st century.

As our attention is now directed to the most powerful refracting surface of the human eye, the cornea, surgeons are embracing the techniques of astigmatic keratotomy with cataract surgery to finally achieve emmetropia. With many surgical approaches to cataract surgery available today, which procedure should the surgeon select to optimize the best uncorrected visual result for the patient? Astigmatic keratotomy uniquely remains the only surgical technique now available for correcting astigmatic refractive errors—until such time when toric intraocular lenses ultimately become available. But how do you create the incisions? Where should the incisions be situated? And what technique should you use?

This text will present a tailor-made approach to cataract extraction combined with arcuate astigmatic keratotomy using a "minimal touch" technique for the simultaneous correction of pre-existing astigmatic refractive errors at the time of cataract surgery. This textbook will assume that the surgeon has learned, and mastered well, the many advances in cataract surgical technique of the last decade of the 20th century. Namely, the surgeon should be familiar with the use of topical anesthesia, clear-corneal incision construction, phacoemulsification, capsulorhexis, hydrodissection and small-incision intraocular lenses (IOLs). The surgeon should be comfortable enough with small incisions and one-handed surgical technique to successfully perform these surgical maneuvers with minimal contact with the eye.

To neutralize pre-existing astigmatism, the surgeon must accurately measure what is present preoperatively. This, too, assumes that careful, preoperative retinoscopy has been performed measuring both the power and the axis of the plus cylinder. In addition, computer-assisted video keratography (topography) is a must. The color maps generated by this device are the guide to accurate astigmatic correction. Not all astigmatic cylinders are symmetrical. Many exist at more than one axis. Heretofore, this has been impossible to determine without corneal topography. Performing careful astigmatic surgery without a topographic map is analogous to driving a car at night without headlights—most of the time you can go straight, but eventually you will run into something. Preoperative myopic and hyperopic refractive errors can be corrected with careful and accurate ultrasonic biometry, and selection of the intraocular lens power to achieve emmetropia. As you will see later in this text, arcuate keratotomy incisions do not alter corneal circumference, and therefore, have a minimal effect on the total refractive power of the cornea. Because of this, intraocular lens power need not be changed to compensate for a change in astigmatism correction following the arcuate astigmatic keratotomy.

The purpose of the eye is to refract light and create a clear image for the brain. The cornea and the lens make up the most important components of the refractive system of the eye. Just as removing a human crystalline lens (cataract extraction) without replacing it with an artificial lens (IOL implantation) is leaving the eye in the worst refractive condition (aphakia), so is the removal of a cataract combined with lens implantation without correcting the pre-existing refractive state of the eye to achieve emmetropia. Essentially this is concentrating on the route while ignoring the destination. Our goal of modern ocular microsurgery is to leave the eye in a better refractive state at the end of a surgical procedure than it was before surgery. Ultimately, isn't that what we want for our patients, for them to see better? To achieve this, we may need to replace a clouded natural lens with a clear artificial lens, correct pre-existing astigmatism with keratotomy, and eliminate myopia, hyperopia, and presbyopia with correctly powered IOLs. To perform a cataract extraction without paying attention to these goals is irresponsible given today's technological advances.

The authors of this textbook are in agreement that a unified approach to cataract surgery with the simultaneous permanent correction of astigmatic, hyperopic, myopic, and presbyopic refractive errors is needed. Through remodeling the cornea and the lens simultaneously (keratolenticuloplasty), surgeons can utilize keratorefractive procedures and lens replacement surgery to correct all forms of refractive errors. Surgeons should not only learn these techniques, but make them a regular part of their practice. This textbook will show you how.

Chapter 1

The Physiological Basis of Refraction

Robert M. Kershner, MD, FACS

The human eye is a compound optical system. The most powerful refracting portion is the cornea and the lens. Light rays entering the eye are refracted most strongly as they pass from air to the corneal density at the surface of the cornea. The cornea is responsible for almost 80% of the refractive power of the eye. The crystalline lens then focuses the remaining power, with the axial length controlling the refractive error.

Gullstrand, at the turn of the century, developed an optical model of the eye which is composed of six spherical refracting surfaces; two for the cornea and four for the crystalline lens (Figure 1-1). Of this system, the corneal refracting power and the length of the eye are the two most powerful elements in determining the refractive state. Light rays which fall short of the retina create a myopic state (Figure 1-2). Light rays which fall in focus behind the retina create a hyperopic state (Figure 1-3). Corneal topography demonstrates the steeper regions of the cornea which can bend the light more strongly preventing a single point of focus on the retina, known as astigmatism (Figure 1-4).

For the purposes of discussion, we are going to assume that myopic, hyperopic, and eventually presbyopic refractive states can be corrected by careful selection of the power and type of the intraocular lens implant. The most important component of this formulation, axial length of the eye, can be measured by precise ultrasonic biometry, and appropriate IOL selection. We are left then, with the need to correct the irregularities in the refracting power of the cornea.

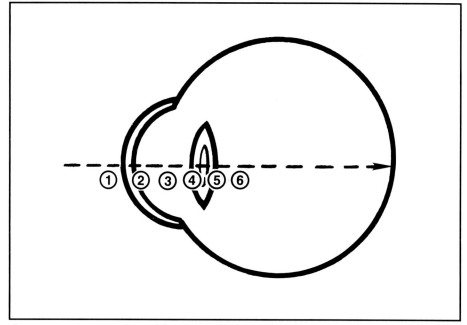

Figure 1-1. Refracting surfaces of the eye. The cornea and the axial length are the most significant.

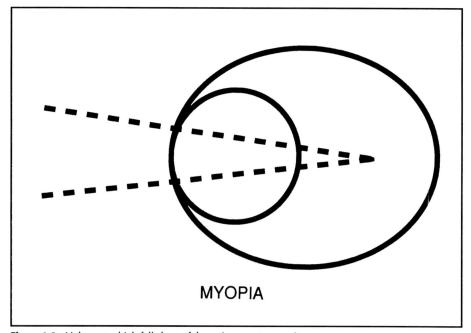

Figure 1-2. Light rays which fall short of the retina create myopia.

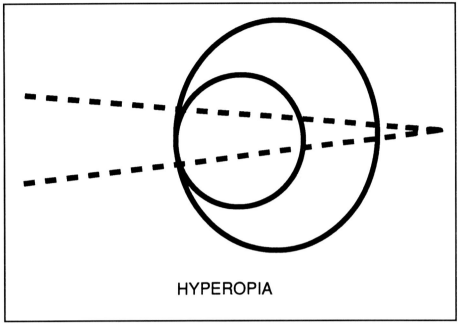

HYPEROPIA

Figure 1-3. Light rays which focus beyond the retina create hyperopia.

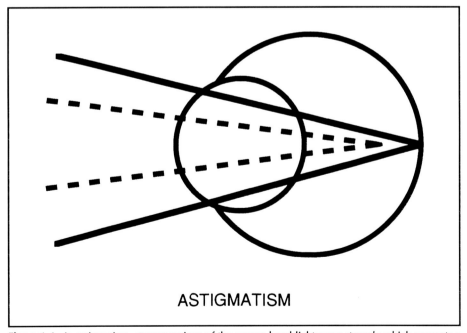

ASTIGMATISM

Figure 1-4. In astigmatism, steeper regions of the cornea bend light more strongly which prevents a single point of focus.

Why should surgeons concern themselves at all with the correction of corneal astigmatism? Can't a properly prescribed cylinder in a spectacle lens do the same thing without all the extra work? The answer rests with the fact that the cylinder in a spectacle lens produces distortion due to meridional aniseikonia. The unequal magnification of the retinal image in various meridians can create intolerable symptoms for the patient. This occurs only under binocular conditions. Even minor degrees of monocular distortion from astigmatism can produce large degrees of binocular spatial aberrations in perception. This is perceived by the patient as tilting lines or altered shapes of objects. The only means we have available for treating binocular spatial distortion is by correcting the monocular distortion which produces it. Surgeons must appreciate this concept to understand why a patient who can otherwise see 20/20 with correction may be terribly unhappy with the surgical result if residual astigmatism is present. By leaving the patient with as close to a spherical cornea as possible at the end of the surgical procedure, the risk of inducing optical distortion is reduced and the result is a happier patient.

The cornea is a complex though predictable architectural structure. Its refracting power is dependent upon a clear tear film, smooth epithelial surface, and lack of opacities or irregularities in the media. The average width of the human cornea is 12.5 mm horizontally, and 11.5 mm vertically. Although the cornea is round when viewed from behind, it is ovoid when viewed from the front due to the encroachment onto the corneal surface of the limbus. In fact, the optical center of the cornea is approximately 5.2 mm from the superior limbus and 6.23 mm from the temporal limbus. That is why temporal corneal incisions are further from the optical center of the eye than superiorly placed incisions (Figure 1-5).

The strength of the cornea is in the Descemet's membrane. The epithelium, Bowman's membrane, and the regular array of collagen fibers that constitute the stroma all contribute to the structural integrity of the cornea to a much lesser degree. Because of this microanatomical structure, we can alter corneal curvature without substantially affecting its strength.

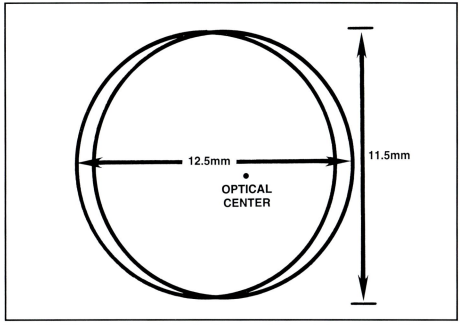

Figure 1-5. Right eye showing optical center of cornea and distance to temporal corneal limbus.

Corneal Incisions

All latitudinally placed corneal incisions, like the latitude lines on a globe, reduce the corneal curvature in that meridian, and therefore, flatten it. Latitudinal incisions have no effect on corneal circumference, and therefore, unlike radial incisions, have no effect on the net power of the cornea. This basic principle can be used to our advantage when preferentially flattening steeper areas as in the correction of corneal astigmatism. Straight transverse incisions are not as effective in altering corneal curvature. A straight line on a sphere is, in fact, a reverse curve or a frown. As the straight transverse incision traverses the corneal dome, it travels from thinner to thicker cornea, and therefore, is unequal in depth. Arcuate incisions, in contrast, are equal in depth as they closely parallel the optical zone and remain within the same latitude of corneal thickness (Figure 1-6). By varying the proximity of the arcuate incision to the optical center of the cornea, and by varying its length, its net effect on the refractive power of the cornea in that meridian can be controlled. The depth of the incision should always remain constant, and should be no less than 85% corneal thickness, and no more than 95% in depth. Experience has shown that arcuate keratotomy incisions should not

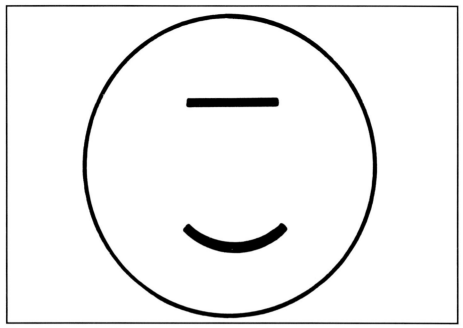

Figure 1-6. Arcuate incisions, unlike straight transverse incisions, are equal in depth by paralleling the optical zone at a given corneal thickness.

approach closer than the 5-mm optical zone to avoid visual effects of glare. By comparison, incisions at the 5-mm optical zone will exert more refractive effect for a given length than incisions closer to the limbus. When choosing an optical zone, the amount of refractive effect should be balanced against the increased symptoms caused by having the incision closer to the optical center of the eye, and therefore, more likely to cause visual aberration due to the defraction of light. Similar length arcuate incisions from the 5-mm optical zone to the 9-mm optical zone will correspondingly exert less refractive effect as they are placed in thicker cornea and further from the optical center of the eye. In most instances, it is preferable to use a slightly longer arcuate incision at a larger optical zone than a smaller incision closer to the optical center of the cornea. Some surgeons advocate keeping all arcuate incisions within the 7-mm optical zone. This increases the simplicity of calculations, and reduces the instrumentation required. However, it forces the surgeon to utilize larger arcuate incisions to gain greater astigmatic effects. If the surgeon is contemplating utilizing an arcuate keratotomy incision for the cataract procedure, the incision at an optical zone of 7 mm is undesirable. I advocate a range of optical zones from 5 mm to 9 mm to provide surgeons with the greatest flexibility. Arcuate corneal incisions greater than 60°, with a chord

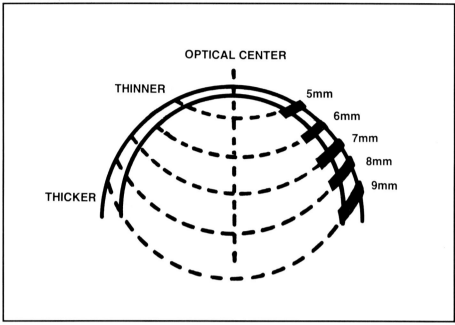

Figure 1-7. Arcuate keratotomy incisions placed at varying optical zones.

length of approximately 4 mm, should be avoided (Figure 1-7). Arcuate keratotomy incisions can be expressed in degrees of arc much like looking at a protractor. They also can be expressed in the chord length of that incision. Generally speaking, each 15° of arc at a 7-mm optical zone represents approximately 1 mm in chord length (Figure 1-8). I find, in teaching the techniques of arcuate astigmatic keratotomy, that surgeons have difficulty thinking in degrees. Therefore, I personally prefer measuring incisions in millimeters of chord length.

The benefits of the arcuate keratotomy incision can be combined with its ability to flatten corneal curvature in the meridian in which it is placed. I advocate, therefore, the use of an *arcuate incision for cataract surgery*. This incision can start at the clear cornea, just anterior to the vascular arcade at the limbus. Its length can range from 5.0 mm for single piece PMMA IOLs to 2.0 mm for small elastic injectable IOLs (Figure 1-9). The length of the arcuate incision placed at the limbus (9.0-mm to 10.0-mm optical zone) will correspondingly induce a certain degree of flattening. This flattening can be measured, and is predictable. Longer arcuate limbal incisions placed in the cornea will therefore have greater astigmatic inducing (or neutralizing) effect than shorter arcuate incisions. The correction of larger degrees of astigmatism, when a small (less than 3.0 mm) chord length arcuate incision is

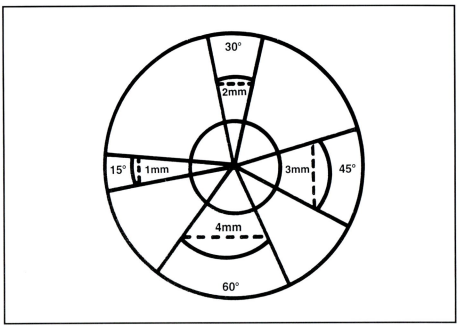

Figure 1-8. An illustration of arcuate incisions at a 7-mm optical zone; 15° = chord length of 1 mm, 30° = chord length of 2 mm, 45° = chord length of 3 mm, and 60° = chord length of 4 mm.

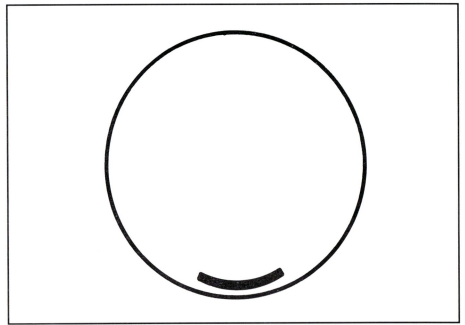

Figure 1-9. A limbal arcuate keratolenticuloplasty incision. The length can be varied for refractive effect and to accomodate the phacoemulsification tip and IOL.

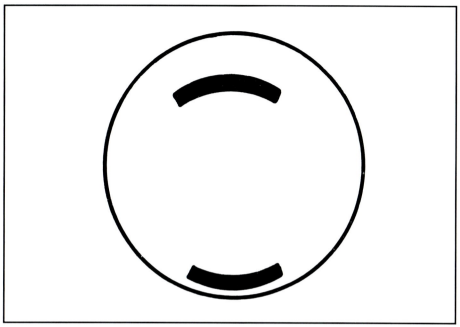

Figure 1-10. A limbal arcuate keratolenticuloplasty incision paired with an arcuate keratotomy incision for maximal astigmatic correction.

utilized, will require the simultaneous pairing of an additional arcuate incision to further neutralize the pre-existing astigmatism (Figure 1-10). By creating an arcuate keratotomy incision for the subsequent stages of cataract removal and pairing it with an arcuate incision for maximum refractive effect, the surgeon is provided with the greatest flexibility in correcting all forms of pre-existing astigmatism (Figure 1-11).

Constructing the Arcuate Keratotomy Incision

There are several diamond keratomes available for creating corneal incisions. Most radial keratotomy, as well as cataract keratomes, are not ideal for creating the arcuate incision. The ideal diamond keratome is a square-edged diamond (Figure 1-12A). When placed into the substance of the cornea and gently rotated in the direction of the incision, an equal depth arcuate keratotomy can be created which is squared off at each edge. With practice, back-cutting diamonds (Figure 1-12B), and bidirectional diamond keratomes (Figure 1-12C) can be used in a similar fashion.

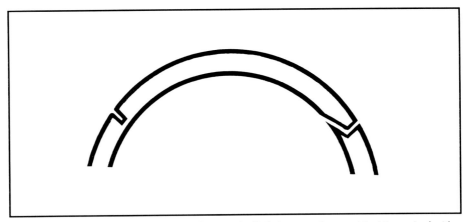

Figure 1-11. Cross-section of Figure 1-10 showing the limbal arcuate (cataract) incision paired with a refractive arcuate keratotomy. The length of the arc, proximity to the optical zone and axis can be varied depending upon the power of astigmatism.

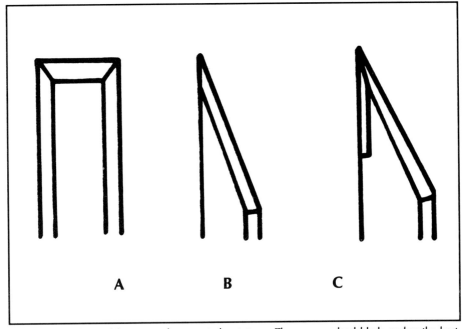

Figure 1-12. Diamond keratomes for arcuate keratotomy. The square-edged blade makes the best, equal-depth, squared-off incision (A). Other blades are the back-cutting (B) and bidirectional-cutting (C) blades.

Because of the oblique angle of the cutting surface, these blades will tend to swim in the stroma of the cornea, and the arcuate incision will not be smooth. In addition, the non-square edged keratome will not square off the ends of the incision.

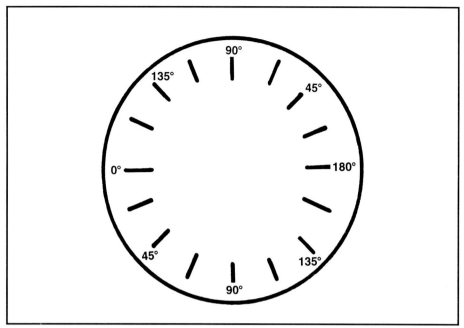

Figure 1-13. The operating microscope astigmatic reticle as seen through the objective eye piece.

The accurate axis of the astigmatism to be corrected can be matched by using a reticule in the microscope (Figure 1-13). Once the arcuate keratotomies are created, the incision closest to the surgeon can be utilized for the cataract procedure. A tri-faceted keratome is placed perpendicular to the base of the incision and a 1.25 mm track into clear cornea is created. The surgeon can then complete the cataract surgery.

The creation of arcuate keratotomy incisions can be one of the most demanding, though powerful, surgical techniques in a surgeon's hands. Understanding the foundation in which this technology is based is crucial to accurately applying it. Take the time now to review the corneal anatomy, the basics of corneal curvature, and how this technique affects refractive power before proceeding with the various techniques in which it will be put to use.

Chapter 2

Incisional Keratotomy
Effects on Corneal Curvature and Refractive Power of the Eye

Spencer P. Thornton, MD, FACS

Modern incisional keratotomy was introduced to the United States in 1978 by Svyatoslav Fyodorov of Russia and Leo Bores of the United States. Since that time there has been a revolution in the treatment of myopia and astigmatism. Paralleling this revolution has been the quieter revolution in the technology of intraocular lenses and the approach to cataract surgery, with the major advances represented by phacoemulsification, small incision surgery and continuous tear capsulotomy (capsulorhexis).

With the potential for astigmatism-neutral cataract surgery provided by recent technological advances in wound architecture, the progressive surgeon has looked for ways to correct pre-existing and postoperative abnormalities of corneal curvature. In addition to changes in position of the cataract incision to produce flattening of that meridian, it is natural that he should look to incisional refractive surgery for further astigmatic correction.

An understanding of the refractive changes produced by incisional keratotomy will aid us in realizing the potential for providing emmetropia to astigmatic corneas during and after the cataract procedure. We shall first look at the theoretical basis for corneal curvature changes with corneal relaxing incisions (CRIs).

The Tissue Relaxation Principle

When tissue is removed from the cornea (as by wedge resection), the radius of curvature is reduced, the curvature steepened and the refractive power increased. When tissue is added to the cornea the radius of curvature is increased, the curvature flattened and the refractive power reduced (Figure 2-1). All incisions act as if tissue is added.

An unsutured incision in the cornea relaxes tissue and increases the circumference. The tissue is "added" or "relaxed" at right angles to the direction of the incision (Figure 2-2). If the incision is placed radially, its action is transmitted 360° around the circumference of the cornea. In the usual RK, the first incision (and the second incision, if opposite the first) increases the circumference 360° (Figure 2-3).

An incision placed 90° away from the first and second incisions (i.e. halfway between the first and second incisions) acts over an area of 180° (i.e. 90° to either side of that incision) until it hits the previously placed incisions which, because they are in the same relative direction around the periphery or the cornea (i.e. radial to the center of the cornea and perpendicular to the limbus), act as a "relay station," enhancing and reinforcing the effect of each similar incision (Figure 2-4). Any subsequently added incisions have their main action between adjacent incisions (Figure 2-5). Though each additional

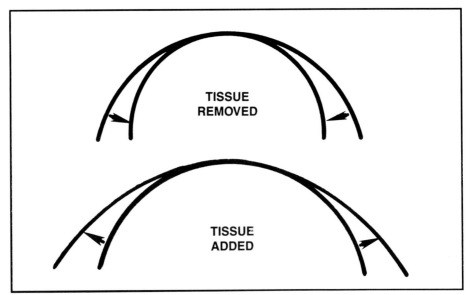

Figure 2-1. Corneal power is changed by removing or adding tissue.

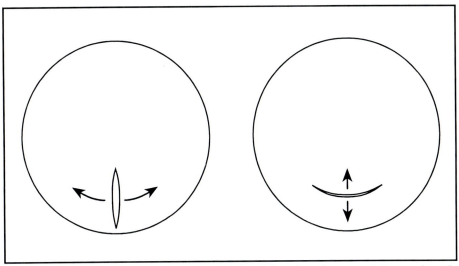

Figure 2-2. Relaxing incisions act as if tissue is added, and the radius of curvature is increased at right angles to the incision.

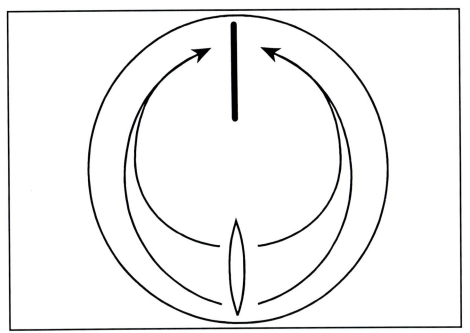

Figure 2-3. Circumference increased 360° by opposing radials with reinforcing effect.

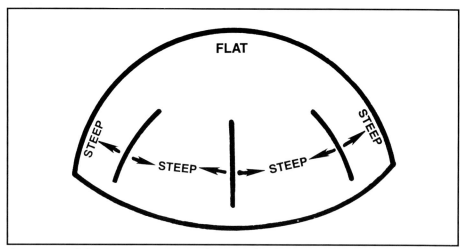

Figure 2-4. Radial incisions increase circumference and each incision reinforces the others.

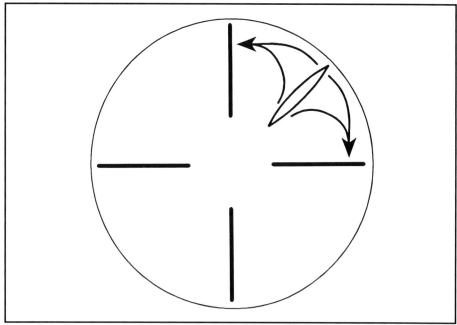

Figure 2-5. The main effect of incisions is between "barriers."

incision increases the effect of previous incisions (if parallel to each other), there is a diminishing effect with each additional incision placed. With radial incisions the effect is as shown in Table 2-1.

Table 2-1.
Relative Effect of RK Incisions in 8 Incision RK

Incision	% of Total Effect
1	20 - 25%
2	35 - 45%
3	50 - 55%
4	60 - 65%
5	70 - 75%
6	80 - 85%
7	90 - 95%
8	100%

Barrier Tissue and the "Barrier" Effect

Previously unaltered or "virgin" corneal tissue is congruous and acts as a uniform transmitter of curvature change produced by any force applied to it internally or externally. In fact, any congruous tissue transmits forces of relaxation or tension uniformly unless impaired in some way. If there is any interference by a "barrier" or discontinuity, this uniformity will be interrupted. Tissues noncongruous to the corneal stroma are the limbus and any scars which may be present in the cornea.

Another incision crossing the path of the area altered by an incision also acts as a barrier. This barrier may impede the effect or enhance it depending on the direction of the incision. When that incision is in the same direction (as with additional radial incisions) the effect is enhanced between the incisions. When the incision is at right angles to the primary incision the effect is impeded or restricted (as in the case of combined "T" incisions and radials)(Figure 2-6).

Since tissue is effectively added with any incision, no matter what its curvature, or lack of it, the "added tissue" is at right angles to the incision, and in the meridian of steep curvature across the corneal dome the resulting increase in circumference is limited by the limbus to a "band" across the

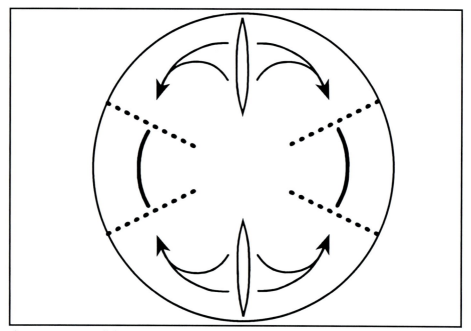

Figure 2-6. Nonparallel incisions restrict effect. The "barrier" zone is indicated by the dots.

cornea—the meridional corneal diameter. The limbus thus acts as a "barrier" and confines the effect of the relaxing incisions primarily to the area between the incisions (Figure 2-7), much as a megaphone magnifies sound confined within the walls of the megaphone.

Transverse Incisions

Transverse relaxing incisions, whether straight "T" incisions or arcuate incisions, "add tissue" in the meridian across which they are placed (remember, the action produced by an incision is at right angles to the incision). The reason these incisions are so powerful is that their circumferential effect is restricted and concentrated by a "limiting barrier," the limbus (see Figure 2-7).

This confining of the effect of arcuate incisions acts to magnify the effect, and accounts for the fact that these incisions are so powerful for any given length. We have found clinically that up to 2.5 diopters of astigmatism can be

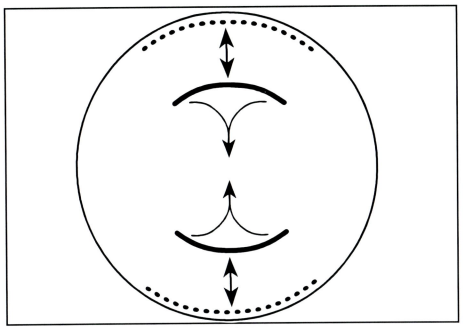

Figure 2-7. The limbal barrier confines the effect of relaxing incisions.

corrected with only one arcuate incision across the steep meridian (on the steeper side as indicated by corneal topography), aiming at slight under-correction.

Coupling

Whereas radial incisions increase the circumference of the peripheral cornea as they relax tissue around the circumference, *transverse* incisions, if placed parallel to the limbus and concentric to the center of the visual axis, relax only the meridian in which they are placed and do not increase the corneal circumference. If there is no increase in the circumference of the cornea a phenomenon called "coupling" occurs. Coupling is the effect of incisions that relax and flatten the steeper meridian to steepen the flatter meridian 90° away (Figure 2-8). The coupling effect of transverse incisions is offset or reduced by added radial incisions or transverse incisions which are so long as to become semiradial.

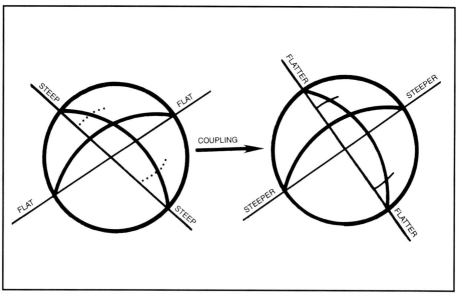

Figure 2-8. Illustration of the concept of "coupling."

Straight Versus Arcuate Incisions

It is difficult to depict a three-dimensional concept with a two-dimensional illustration, and because transverse incisions have been depicted in presentations and published papers as straight lines, the potential of coupling has not been fully realized (Figure 2-9).

All straight lines on a spherical surface are curved and straight transverse incisions are actually inverse arcs and are therefore semiradial. The longer the incision the more radial it becomes. Concentric arcuate incisions on the other hand are parallel to the equator (the limbus) and transverse to the meridian and therefore have greater effect on the meridian transversed.

Arcuate incisions, precisely following the curve of the circular optical zone, have the potential for greater effect because the chord length is the same as straight transverse incisions, but the actual length is about 10% longer on the curve and the entire length of the incision is at the calculated optical zone.

The difficulty in producing precise, reproducible concentric arcuate incisions has chiefly been because of instrumentation. The diamond blades used for radial and transverse corneal incisions have been relatively wide (either 1 mm square tipped or angled from 35° to 45°), making curved incisions difficult. The new "triple edged arcuate" diamond blade with its 200μ square cutting tip overcomes this difficulty (Figure 2-10).

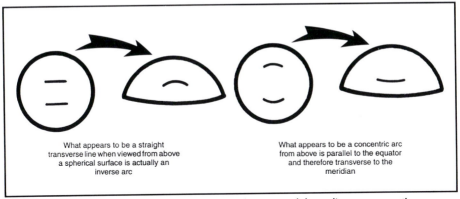

What appears to be a straight
transverse line when viewed from above
a spherical surface is actually an
inverse arc

What appears to be a concentric arc
from above is parallel to the equator
and therefore transverse to the
meridian

Figure 2-9. Lines on a spherical surface appear straight or curved depending on perspective.

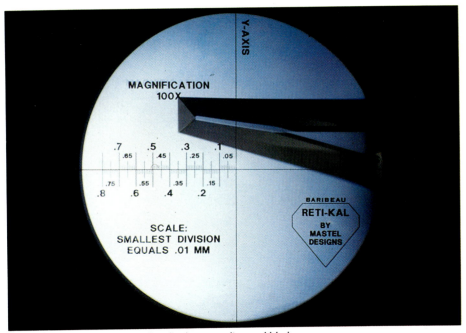

Figure 2-10. The Thornton Triple-Edged arcuate diamond blade.

Inverse Arc Incisions

Taking the concept of arcuate incisions a step further, it can be demonstrated that an exaggerated inverse arc (Figure 2-11) can flatten the steep meridian and at the same time increase the peripheral circumference, reducing myopia. This has its greatest use in cases of myopic astigmatism in

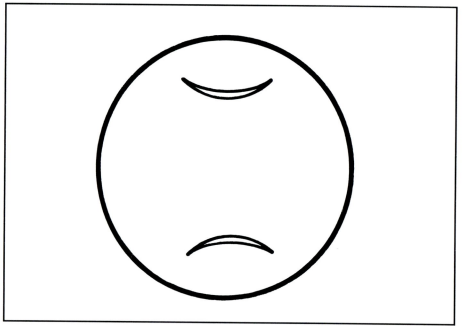

Figure 2-11. Inverse arc incisions.

which a reduction of the myopic spherical equivalent, otherwise produced by arcuate incisions, is desired without having to place additional radial incisions. You can *reduce the induced myopic spherical equivalent by one half the amount of the cylinder corrected by using inverse arc incisions.*

Summary

The goal of emmetropia with cataract surgery is now attainable even in cases of high pre-existing astigmatism because of the advances in instrumentation and technique of incisional keratotomy which can be performed at the time of cataract surgery. Nomograms are available for accurate, predictable astigmatic keratotomy which are as reliable as those for calculation of intraocular lens power, and courses in incisional keratotomy are available on an ever increasing basis.

Chapter 3

Keratolenticuloplasty

Robert M. Kershner, MD, FACS

Cataract surgery has undergone a phenomenal change in the past ten years. At one time in-patient hospitalization, general anesthesia, large surgical incisions, multiple sutures, and aphakic spectacle correction postoperatively were the norm. Gradually, cataract surgeons improved cataract removal techniques allowing better visual rehabilitation with intraocular lens implantation. Careful selection of small incision one-piece and three-piece IOLs made IOL implantation possible without significantly altering astigmatism. In time, surgical techniques evolved from large incision extracapsular extraction with sutures to sutureless small incision phacoemulsification, minimizing iatrogenically-induced astigmatism from the procedure. With each incremental change, cataract surgery has evolved towards our ultimate goal of complete visual restoration—acuity unencumbered by corrective lenses. Pre-existing refractive errors including astigmatism and presbyopia, however, continue to persist as the leading indication for postoperative spectacle correction.

Spherical errors are correctable with careful and accurate preoperative ultrasonic biometry and appropriate intraocular lens selection. In the near future, presbyopia may be correctable with an intraocular lens implant with bifocal capability. However, pre-existing astigmatic errors continue to plague the cataract surgeon. Although small incision surgery has reduced the postoperative iatrogenic astigmatism, the smaller incisions have less ability to tailor pre-existing astigmatism. Recent advances in the corneal approach to cataract surgery have created the opportunity for the surgeon to take advantage of the corneal incision placement to fully correct the refractive error of the patient at the time of cataract extraction. This creates new opportunities to improve uncorrected visual acuity postoperatively. I have named the procedure for remodeling the cornea with refractive keratotomy and replacing the lens through the same incision—keratolenticuloplasty (KLP).

There are compelling reasons to fully correct all refractive errors at the time of surgery. First, is patient preference and lifestyle. Freedom to be able to drive, work, read, swim, and play without dependence on spectacle or contact lenses is a normal desire. Second is economic. In the United States alone over three billion dollars a year is spent on eyewear (glasses and contact lenses). Eliminating dependence on these appliances will save the consumer hundreds of millions of dollars in doctor's visits, refractions, fitting and dispensing of eyewear.

The number one refractive procedure performed in the United States today is cataract surgery. Therefore, all cataract surgeons are in fact already refractive surgeons. The recent advances in the technology of computer-assisted videokeratography (corneal topography), finely calibrated keratomes for corneal incisions, and precision methods of measuring corneal thickness (ultrasonic pachymetry) have provided the refractive surgeon with superior tools for achieving precise and reproducible refractive corrections. Today, as ophthalmic surgeons, we have the ability to correct all forms of refractive errors. To do any less for our patients is to miss a golden opportunity of satisfying one of mankinds lifelong desires—normal vision.

Keratolenticuloplasty—The Procedure

Surgeons should be wary of those who claim that they perform one cataract incision technique "100% of the time." There is no single approach to cataract surgery which is ideal for all patients. Today's technological advances and instrumentation allow us to use a "tailor-made" approach to surgery. Surgeons who are undertaking refractive cataract surgery should be well versed in small-incision cataract surgery, capsulorhexis, hydrodissection, in-the-bag phacoemulsification and small incision intraocular lens implantation.[1-3] Knowledge and use of topical anesthesia is helpful, although not mandatory.

The key to this procedure is careful preoperative keratometry of the cornea. It is important to perform meticulous ultrasonic biometry to determine the proper spherical correction to be provided by the intraocular lens implant. To purposefully undercorrect or overcorrect a given refractive error (i.e., to match the other eye or to maintain the preoperative refractive error) is absurd. The surgeon should aim for emmetropia with no residual postoperative refractive error at all times.

A complete examination of the eye should always be performed. Attention to the cornea to screen for scarring, epithelial defects, irregularities, or guttata is important. A cycloplegic refraction and recording of the preoperative astigmatic error is crucial. Computerized topography enables the surgeon to identify the axis of steepest astigmatism (which sometimes may be quite asymmetrical) and should be performed if at all possible. A surgical plan can then be developed.

Careful incision construction is the key to a self-sealing and rapidly healing incision. The anatomy and architecture of scleral-tunnel and clear-corneal incisions have been discussed extensively elsewhere.[3-6] Sutureless scleral-tunnel incisions can be almost completely astigmatically neutral in that they do not induce iatrogenic astigmatism. They are, however, incapable of correcting pre-existing astigmatism. Clear-corneal incisions, properly constructed, can be minimally astigmatic. Arcuate corneal incisions which parallel the optical zone induce the most flattening. Straight transverse incisions induce less flattening and reverse curve (frown) incisions induce the least. The incision's tendency to alter corneal curvature can be utilized to correct pre-existing astigmatic errors. Clear-corneal incisions can be combined with an arcuate keratotomy to maximize the astigmatic correcting potential of the incision.

The basics of arcuate corneal incisions have been well described by Dr. Spencer Thornton and others,[7-9] and can be reviewed elsewhere in this text. Arcuate corneal incisions exert greater effect for less surgery because they exactly follow the radius of the optical zone. Arcuate incisions have the same chord length as simple straight transverse incisions. However, they exert about 20% greater effect in changing corneal curvature than straight incisions. I therefore use only arcuate incisions for the correction of astigmatism and make all transverse corneal incisions (cataract, astigmatic, etc.) as arcuate incisions.

I classify cataract incisions into three categories:

1. *Scleral-tunnel incisions*—these incisions are effective when no pre-existing astigmatism is present, and the surgeon does not want to risk changing corneal curvature. They require conjunctival dissection, and cautery, and are not ideal when future filtering procedures are contemplated.

2. *Single clear-corneal incisions*—single arcuate keratotomy incisions at the 9.0-mm or 10.0-mm optical zone can be strategically positioned to correct small degrees of pre-existing astigmatism.

3. *Paired arcuate keratotomy incisions*—for the correction of larger degrees of pre-existing astigmatism, the arcuate keratotomy incision for cataract surgery can be paired with an additional arcuate incision on the opposite end of the same meridian.

There is some debate over whether astigmatic keratotomy should be performed at the start of a cataract procedure, at the conclusion of the cataract procedure, or at a later date following the surgery. As clear-corneal surgery fails to alter pre-existing refractive errors unless purposely created to do so, it makes little sense to wait until a later date. When given the opportunity to have their refractive error corrected at the time of cataract surgery or as a separate procedure, 100% of the patients in my practice opt for the single procedure. Waiting until after the eye is healed from cataract surgery made sense at one time when the postoperative refractive error was unpredictable, but makes little sense today with self-sealing and rapidly healing incisions of less than 3.0 mm.

I also feel it makes no sense to place an incision on the sclera for cataract surgery only to make two transverse incisions for the correction of residual astigmatism (the so-called TAK procedure). If the surgeon needs to make an access for the steps of the cataract surgery, it makes more sense to purposefully place that incision to take full advantage of its astigmatically neutralizing (flattening) effect. Hence, the concept of the arcuate keratotomy incision for cataract surgery (KLP) was born.

When the preoperative astigmatic cylinder exceeds one diopter, a single arcuate clear-corneal keratotomy is utilized for the cataract incision (Table 3-1). Astigmatic powers greater than 1.50 D can be corrected with a combined approach of a clear-corneal arcuate keratotomy and a paired arcuate keratotomy opposite the cataract incision. The incisions are placed to correspond to the steepest axis of astigmatism at each meridian on either side of the optical zone as determined by preoperative topography. In many instances, the axis of astigmatism is not symmetrical and, therefore, the arcuate incisions are positioned to correspond to the steepest axis of each arm of the astigmatism. Arcuate incisions are placed from 2.5 mm to 5.0 mm from the optical center of the cornea according to nomograms for the correction desired (in diopters). In most cases of keratolenticuloplasty, either a single 2.5-mm or 3.0-mm arcuate keratotomy at the 8-mm to 10-mm optical zone or

Table 3-1.
Kershner Arcuate Keratotomy System
Nomograms

Correction (Diopters)	Optical Zone (mm)	Arcuate Incision Length (mm)
<1.0	10	2.5 (1)
1.0	9	2.5 (1)
1.5	9	3.0 (1)
2.0	8	2.5 (2)
2.5	9 / 7	2.5 (2)
3.0	9 / 7	3.0 (2)
3.5	8 / 7	3.0 (2)
4.0	6	2.0 (2)
4.5	6	2.5 (2)
5.0	6	3.0 (2)
5.5	5	2.0 (2)
6.0	5	2.5 (2)

Corrected for age 60 +. Arcs placed on steepest axis of astigmatism (plus cylinder). Pachymetry at incision site, square diamond keratome set to 100% of pachymetry. Mark arcuate incisions and optical zone with Kershner One-Step Marker. Cataract keratotomy at 10 mm, 9 mm, or 8 mm only.

a pair of 2.0-mm, 2.5-mm or 3.0-mm incisions at the 7.0-mm to 8-mm optical zones, will be all that is required.

Surgical Technique

The computerized topographic maps are brought to the operating room and positioned next to the patient. A reticule is installed in the objective ocular of the operating microscope and the microscope positioned precisely perpendicular over the patient's eye. The optical zone is identified by having the patient look directly into the light of the microscope. The axis of the cylinder can then be accurately marked by referencing the topographic map with the microscope reticule. Topical anesthesia is desirable for this step and reduces the chance of error by allowing the patient to fixate the eye accurately.

Intraoperative keratometry may be helpful but is not necessary if the microscope is properly positioned and the topography consulted during the procedure. Some day, we will have real-time topographic imaging which will eliminate any error. But until then, the surgeon should consult the topographic map while performing the corneal incisions. Ultrasonic pachymetry is performed at the site of the planned arcuate keratotomy incisions. The patient is once again asked to look into the microscope light. The optical zone is marked by positioning the Kershner One-Step Arcuate Keratotomy marker (Figures 3-1 and 3-2) and, simultaneously, marking both arcuate incision(s) onto the steepest meridian of the cornea (Figure 3-3). The Rhein triple-edged square diamond keratome (Rhein Medical, Tampa, Florida) is set to 100% of the pachymetry (Figure 3-4) measurement by calibrating it under a microscope. The arcuate incisions are then fashioned with the keratome (Figure 3-5A and 3-5B). The keratome is inserted into one edge of the arcuate mark and the cornea applanated. The length of each incision will correspond to the magnitude of the correction required, as determined in the preoperative plan. A gentle rotation of the keratome handle between the thumb and index finger as the diamond is rotated and pulled clockwise allows the blade to track in an arcuate manner. Two arcuate incisions are then created, with each incision squared off at each edge and achieving 95% depth of cut.

The arcuate incision closest to the surgeon is utilized for the keratotomy into the anterior chamber. A 2.5 mm diamond trifaceted keratome is passed into and positioned perpendicular to the base of the arcuate keratotomy, a

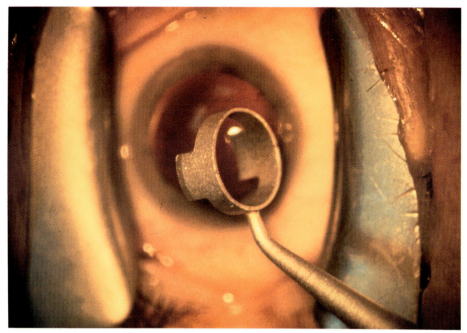

Figure 3-1. Side profile of Kershner arcuate marker.

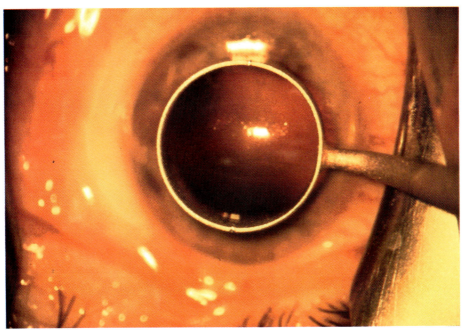

Figure 3-2. The marker is positioned to center the optical zone and the arcs along the steepest axis of astigmatism.

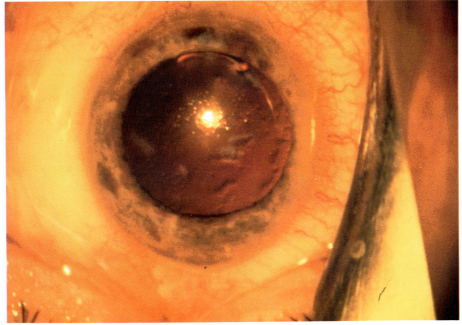

Figure 3-3. Two 3-mm arcuate marks are created.

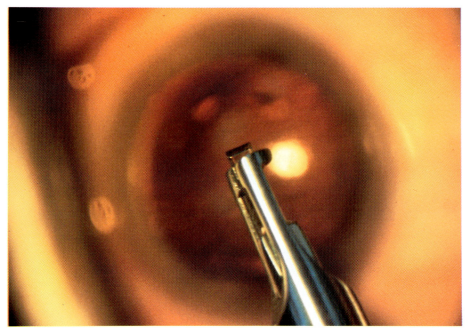

Figure 3-4. The arcuate diamond keratome is set to 100% of pachymetry.

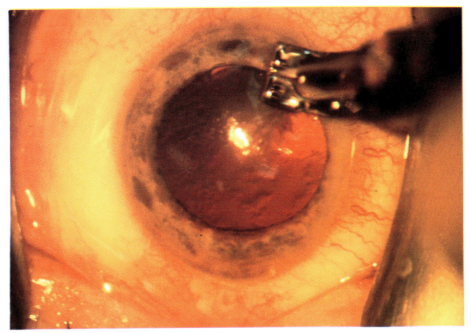

Figure 3-5A.

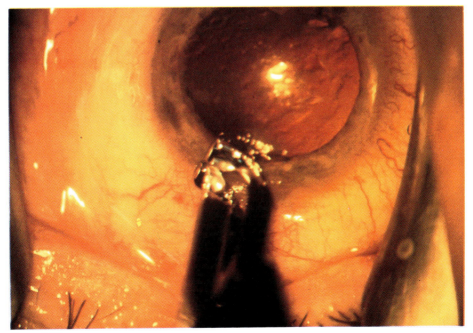

Figure 3-5B.

Figure 3-5. Each arcuate incision is incised.

1.25-mm horizontal corneal track is created at the depth of the arcuate incision (Figure 3-6), and the anterior chamber entered. This leaves approximately 85 microns of tissue at the base of the incision and a 1.25-mm "tunnel" into the anterior chamber. The 2.5-mm keratotomy allows capsulorhexis to be performed with the Kershner cystotome/forceps or with the phaco tip. Hydrodissection and phacoemulsification is then performed and a single-piece silicone IOL such as the STAAR AA4203 is injected into the capsular bag (Figure 3-7). No sutures or bandage contact lenses are used and the eye is not bandaged at the conclusion of the procedure (Figure 3-8). Postoperative antibiotic and anti-inflammatory drops (such as TobraDex, Tobramycin, Dexamethasone solution - Alcon) are started at the conclusion of surgery, and continued four times a day for ten days. The patient is examined at 24 hours, two weeks, three months and at one year.

Figures 3-9 through 3-12 demonstrate the topographic changes induced by clear-corneal incisions and arcuate keratotomy incisions.

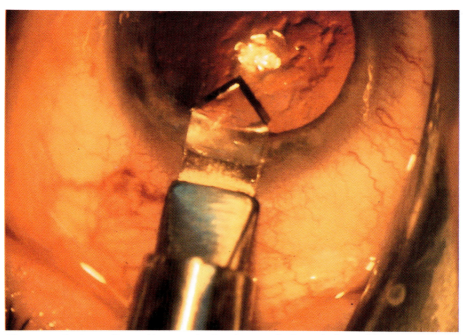

Figure 3-6. A 2.5-mm diamond keratome is placed perpendicular to the base of the arcuate incision closest to the surgeon, entering the anterior chamber 1.25 mm distal to the keratotomy. This creates a two step clear-corneal incision which is self sealing.

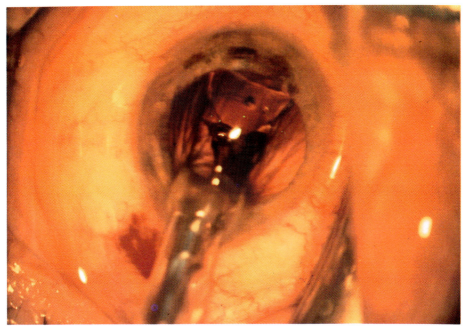

Figure 3-7. A 2.5-mm injection cartridge is used to insert a one-piece elastic lens into the capsular bag.

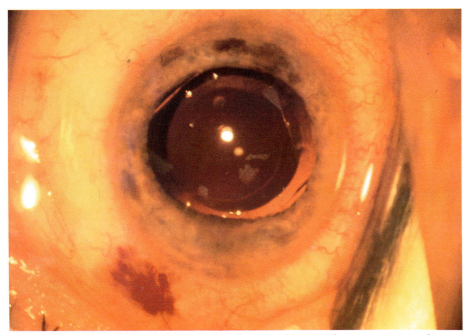

Figure 3-8. The intraocular lens at the conclusion of surgery. The arcuate keratotomy incision does not interfere with visualization.

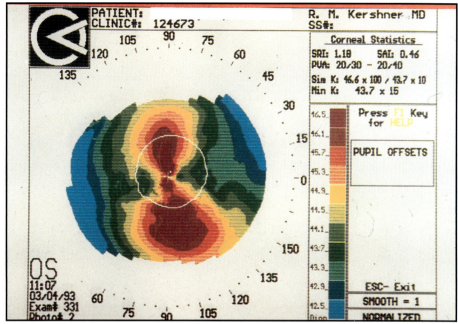

Figure 3-9A. Preoperative topography of with-the-rule astigmatism.

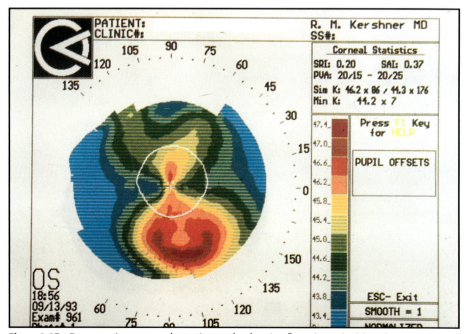

Figure 3-9B. Postoperative topography at six months showing flattening at incision site.

Figure 3-9. Case of with-the-rule astigmatism preoperatively receiving a clear-corneal arcuate incision at 95°.

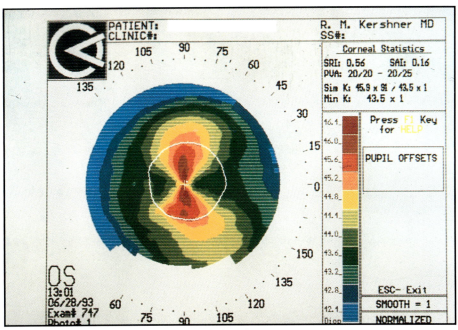

Figure 3-10A. Preoperative topography of with-the-rule astigmatism.

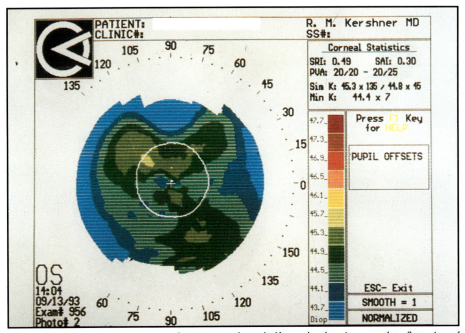

Figure 3-10B. Postoperative topography at two and one-half months showing complete flattening of astigmatism.

Figure 3-10. Case of with-the-rule astigmatism receiving a pair of arcuate keratotomy incisions.

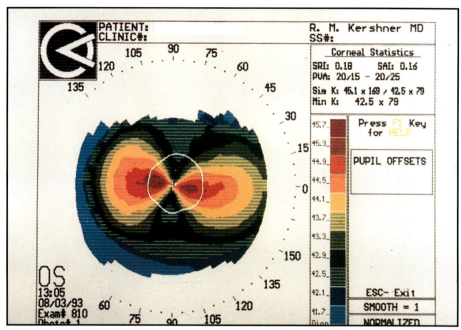

Figure 3-11A. Preoperative topography of against-the-rule astigmatism.

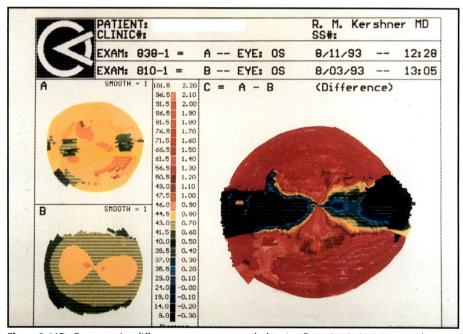

Figure 3-11B. Postoperative difference map at one week showing flattening in incision meridian.

Figure 3-11. Case with against-the-rule astigmatism receiving a pair of arcuate keratotomy incisions.

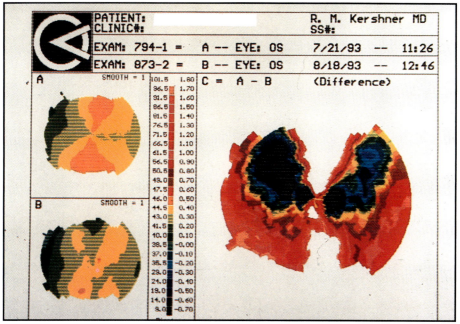

Figure 3-12. Difference map at three weeks postoperatively with paired arcuate incisions at 90°.

Nomogram

When the surgeon elects to perform keratolenticuloplasty, certain rules should be kept in mind. I call these the caveats of KLP.

1. Always slightly undercorrect the pre-existing astigmatism. You can always do more surgery later if needed, but it may be difficult to undo what you have already done if you have done too much. Remember, in older patients, the less elastic cornea responds with greater changes in curvature for a given amount of surgery.

2. It is best to avoid arcuate incisions inside the 7-mm optical zone, unless needed. That is, if it is possible to achieve the same degree of correction at 7 mm with a slightly larger arc, this is to be preferred over a smaller arc at a 6-mm or 5-mm optical zone. In other words, larger incisions are always preferred further away from the optical zone even though their effect decreases as the distance from the optical zone increases.

3. Arcuate incisions should never exceed 60° in length at any optical zone and, ideally, the largest arc should be no greater than 45° or 3 mm.

4. 85% to 95% depth is ideal for an astigmatic effect. Avoid perforating the cornea needlessly, it makes phacoemulsification and maintaining the anterior chamber more difficult.

5. Whenever possible, if a single arcuate incision will suffice, it will be preferable than using two smaller incisions.

6. Always attempt to keep the arcuate incision closest to the surgeon for the keratotomy into the anterior chamber. Place this incision anterior to the limbal vascular arcade at 10 mm, 9 mm or 8 mm. Avoid using the arcuate incision for the subsequent cataract surgery if it is closer to the optical center of the eye than the 8-mm optical zone.

7. To avoid full thickness penetration, avoid pressing on the globe with another instrument during the creation of the arcuate incision. Holding the eye, if required at all, is best performed with a toothed forceps at the conjunctiva. Keep the keratome fully applanated with both footplates and avoid tilting the handle.

8. It is easier to visualize the marks and incise the cornea if the cornea is kept slightly dry.

9. Avoid using marking inks. They obscure visualization for subsequent procedures of cataract surgery. A clean marker gently pressed onto the epithelium will create a visible mark that will be more than satisfactory as a guideline to creating the incision.

10. Simply placing your arcuate corneal cataract incision on the axis of steepest astigmatism will almost always improve the refractive result. However, operating on the incorrect axis will always make the refractive result worse. Axis is crucial. Never operate greater than 15° off axis.

The nomogram (see Table 3-1) is designed to be used with the Kershner One-Step Arcuate Keratotomy system which includes a triple-edge diamond keratome (Rhein Medical - Tampa, Florida, USA) and a set of 3-mm arcuate keratotomy markers with optical zones of 5, 6, 7, 8, and 9 mm. The nomogram is to be used strictly as a guideline. Each individual surgeon should modify his or her values based upon the results obtained in her or his hands.

Summary

Arcuate keratotomy combined with cataract surgery is one of the most powerful techniques we have at present for the permanent correction of pre-existing refractive errors. Take the time to study it carefully and master it well. With experience, it will become one of the most satisfying aspects of your surgical practice.

References

1. Kershner RM: A new one step forceps for capsulorhexis. *J Cataract Refract Surg.* 16:762-767, 1990.

2. Kershner RM: Embryology, anatomy and needle capsulotomy. In Koch PS, Davison JA, eds, *Textbook of Phacoemulsification Techniques*, Thorofare, NJ, SLACK, Inc., pp. 35-48, 1990.

3. Kershner RM: Sutureless one handed intercapsular phacoemulsification - the keyhole technique. *J Cataract Refract Surg.* 17 (supplement):719-725, 1991.

4. Kershner RM: No stitch topical anesthesia. In Gills JP, Hustead RF, Sanders DR, eds, *Ophthalmic Anesthesia*, Thorofare, NJ, SLACK, Inc., pp. 172-175, 1993.

5. Kershner RM: Topical anesthesia for small-incision self-sealing cataract surgery-a prospective study of the first 100 patients. *J Cataract Refract Surg.* 19:290-292, 1993.

6. Kershner RM: Topical anesthesia cataract surgery. In Fine IH, Fichman RA, Grabow HB, eds, *Clear-Corneal Cataract Surgery*, Thorofare, NJ, SLACK, Inc., pp. 141-153, 1993.

7. Rowsey JJ: Review: current concepts in astigmatism surgery. *J Refract Surg.* 2:85-94, 1986.

8. Thornton SP: Astigmatic keratotomy with cataract extraction: Thornton nomogram for quantitative surgery. In Gills JP, Sanders DR, eds, *Small-Incision Cataract Surgery: Foldable Lenses, One-Stitch Surgery, Sutureless Surgery, Astigmatic Keratotomy*, Thorofare, NJ, SLACK, Inc., pp. 245-258, 1990.

9. Thornton SP: Theory behind corneal relaxing incisions/Thornton nomogram. In Gills JP, Martin RG, Sanders DR, eds, *Sutureless Cataract Surgery: An Evolution Toward Minimally Invasive Technique*, Thorofare, NJ, SLACK, Inc., pp. 123-143, 1992.

Chapter 4

Arcuate Keratotomy
for the Correction of Pre-existing and Postcataract Astigmatism

Spencer P. Thornton, MD, FACS

With the safety and efficacy of astigmatic keratotomy well established and the advantages of intraocular lenses long accepted, the aim of the progressive cataract surgeon has become the accomplishment of emmetropia in the postoperative cataract patient.

This is being accomplished in several ways. The architecture of cataract incisions has been improved to the point that surgically induced astigmatism has been markedly reduced. Cataract incisions have become smaller and less astigmatogenic, and the use of scleral pocket three stage incisions and clear-corneal entry has resulted in essentially astigmatism neutral wounds. By proper placement and design of cataract incisions in the steep corneal axis, we have been able to reduce pre-existing astigmatism. But, despite best efforts and advanced techniques, astigmatism associated with cataracts remains a problem. Arcuate keratotomy has been shown to be the most effective means by which pre-existing and postoperative astigmatism can be alleviated.

The question being asked with increased frequency by the progressive cataract surgeon is, "Should I perform corneal relaxing incisions (CRIs) at the time of cataract surgery or wait several months after surgery?" The answer for you as an individual will depend both on your philosophy and the certainty of your astigmatic-neutral cataract surgery.

Astigmatic keratotomy is not a difficult procedure to perform, and, as you will see from the discussion which follows, safe, accurate techniques are within the reach of every skilled ophthalmic surgeon.

When Should Corneal Relaxing Incisions Be Done?

On the one hand, the astigmatic effect of cataract surgery—even with small incisions, and in the best of surgical hands—is sometimes not as accurate as the surgeon would desire, and some postoperative corneal curvature changes can surprise you.

On the other hand, once surgery is performed and excellent vision is achieved with corrective spectacles, especially in patients with large amounts of pre-existing astigmatism, patients are reluctant to undergo another procedure on the same eye and the opportunity to provide emmetropia may be lost. Therefore, increasing numbers of progressive ophthalmologists are studying the theory and principles of corneal relaxing incisions for the correction of pre-existing and postcataract astigmatism.

The question of what to do about pre-existing and surgically induced cylinder has become one of when to do the correction. The answer to this by the progressive ophthalmologist is becoming more and more, "at the time of cataract surgery." The proper techniques of corneal relaxing incisions (AK) are easy to learn, and easily performed.

Prior to incorporating astigmatic keratotomy into your cataract surgical procedure, you must know within a reasonable degree of certainty the refractive result of your cataract incision and wound closure. If you use a 5.0 mm self-sealing superiorly placed wound with 0.75 to 1.25 diopters of against-the rule astigmatic drift between twelve and twenty-four months postoperatively, you can alter the placement of the incision to the temporal cornea and reliably move that astigmatic shift to the horizontal meridian. Many surgeons do just that with good results.

Taking these factors into consideration, astigmatic keratotomy may then be added to further modify the refractive outcome.

Who Are Candidates?

Patients considering cataract surgery who might be considered candidates for astigmatic keratotomy are those with more than 1 D of pre-existing against-the-rule astigmatism or more than 2 D of with-the-rule astigmatism, but the status of the fellow eye must also be carefully evaluated. One should not attempt to remove all against-the-rule astigmatism in one eye when the fellow eye is against-the-rule with good vision, and as a general principle, one should try to leave some with-the-rule astigmatism to compensate for the normal against-the-rule shift with time.

A strong argument can be made that for ultimate accuracy, astigmatic keratotomy should be deferred for several months after cataract surgery so that a stable and precisely known refraction can be used to plan the refractive procedure. But, in the hands of most skilled microsurgeons with modern small incision wounds and foldable intraocular lenses, a significant improvement in results to justify putting the patient through a second, separate procedure is not necessary.

If the decision has been made to perform concomitant astigmatic keratotomy, during the cataract procedure, the decision must be made as to the timing of the placement of corneal relaxing incisions. Some surgeons prefer to place the relaxing incisions prior to the phaco procedure, while others complete the cataract extraction and perform the incisions at the conclusion of the procedure. Similarly, decisions must be made as to when pachymetry must be done, prior to surgery or intraoperatively, and which type of incision is best, straight or arcuate, and with which style blade. For the beginning refractive surgeon, the best way to sort through these questions and to establish a reliable foundation in refractive surgery is to attend a well-known and established radial keratotomy and astigmatic keratotomy course that includes wet-lab instruction.

The preferred technique of this author is to place arcuate relaxing incisions at the conclusion of the cataract procedure after the intraocular lens is in place and the anterior chamber reformed, and the intraocular pressure restored.

In cases in which my cataract incision cannot be easily placed on the steeper meridian, some attempt at vector addition is made to more accurately locate the proper axis for the relaxing incisions. Corneal topography is absolutely essential for this and should be an integral part of the presurgical work-up in any patient in whom astigmatic keratotomy is considered.

Intraoperative keratometry is neither adequate nor accurate in determining incision placement during the cataract procedure.

The correct axis should be determined preoperatively by corneal topography, and carefully marked on the cornea prior to beginning the cataract procedure. A Thornton 360° Arcuate Press-on Marker (Storz) is lightly inked using a pre-inked gentian violet pad (Visitec) and lightly pressed on the dry cornea prior to placing the incisions. This instrument clearly delineates 10° increments of arc at the 6, 7, and 8-mm optical zones. If centering the marker is made difficult by a widely dilated pupil, a small amount of Miochol may be utilized. Intraoperative pachymetry is then performed directly over the planned incision sites. Blade settings are adjusted to achieve an incision depth of 95%.

The Astigmatic Keratotomy Nomogram

The Thornton Nomogram for astigmatic keratotomy is specifically designed to aid the surgeon in determining the precise lengths of arcuate incisions at specific optical zones for reliable and reproducible results in most types of astigmatism (Table 4-1). The nomogram should be carefully followed.

Whereas most nomograms are based on straight incisions of varying lengths at any of several optical zones, a new system for determining arcuate lengths for astigmatic keratotomy has been devised with incision lengths determined in degrees of arc. We are all familiar with the degrees of arc shown on protractors, phoropters and lensometers (Figure 4-1). A 360° press-on

Table 4-1.
Incision Lengths at Varying Optical Zones

Length	5 mm OZ	6 mm OZ	7 mm OZ	8 mm OZ
20°	0.9 mm	1.0 mm	1.2 mm	1.4 mm
25°	1.0 mm	1.3 mm	1.5 mm	1.7 mm
30°	1.3 mm	1.5 mm	1.8 mm	2.0 mm
35°	1.5 mm	1.8 mm	2.1 mm	2.4 mm
40°	1.7 mm	2.0 mm	2.4 mm	2.7 mm
45°	1.9 mm	2.3 mm	2.7 mm	3.1 mm
50°	2.1 mm	2.5 mm	2.9 mm	3.4 mm

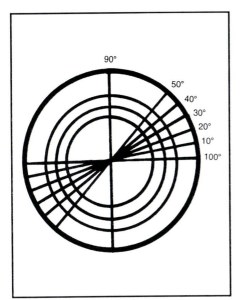

Figure 4-1. A new system for determining arcuate incision lengths for astigmatic keratotomy.

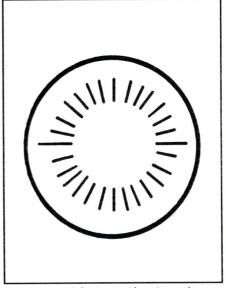

Figure 4-2. 10° divisions with an internal diameter of 6 mm and an external diameter of 8 mm.

corneal marker is now available to give precise arc lengths at the 6, 7, or 8-mm optical zones (Figure 4-2). Specific chord lengths for these arc measurements have been calculated for several optical zones (Table 4-2).

Though arcuate incisions are slightly more difficult to make, they give greater effect with shorter length. With arcuate incisions one can reduce the arc length and increase the number of paired incisions and maximize coupling. With perfect arcuate "T" incisions the coupling is one to one, that is for every diopter of flattening produced in the steep meridian, there is a diopter of steepening produced in the flatter meridian 90° away, keeping the spherical equivalent constant (see Chapter 2). By maximizing coupling in this manner, we do not need to modify our IOL power calculations.

Technique and Instruments

To facilitate the arcuate incision, the "triple edged arcuate diamond" blade is used (Mastel Designs). Fixation is achieved with a Thornton ring. This permits optimal positioning of the globe in that incisional keratotomy is a bimanual technique, and the fixating hand can be used to move the eye

Table 4-2.

Thornton Nomogram for Astigmatic Keratotomy

Assumes cuts 98% deep (almost to Descemet's membrane) along the full length of the incision.
The Sum of the Modifiers = The Theoretical Target Cylinder

Age: For every year below age 30, add ½% to the astigmatic error. For every year above age 30, subtract ½% per year.

Sex: In premenopausal women (under age 40) subtract three years from actual age.

IOP: For every mm IOP below 12, add 2% to cylinder error. For every mm IOP above 15, subtract 2% from amount of cylinder.

Cylinder Corrected by Paired Arcuate Transverse Incisions

Chord Length of One Pair Arcuate Transverse Incisions

Theoretical Cylinder	Degrees Arc
0.50 D	20°
0.75 D	23°
1.00 D	25°
1.25 D	28°
1.50 D	32°
1.75 D	35°
2.00 D	38°
2.25 D	42°
2.50 D	45°

One pair always placed at the 7 mm OZ

Chord Length of Two Pair Arcuate Transverse Incisions

Theoretical Cylinder	Degrees Arc
2.00 D	23°
2.25 D	27°
2.50 D	31°
2.75 D	35°
3.00 D	39°
3.25 D	43°
3.50 D	47°
3.75 D	48°

Two pairs outer at the 8
inner at the 6

Chord Length of Three Pair Arcuate Transverse Incisions

Theoretical Cylinder	Degrees Arc
3.25 D	22°
3.50 D	26°
3.75 D	30°
4.00 D	35°
4.25 D	40°
4.50 D	45°
4.75 D	50°
5.00 D	54°

Three pairs outer just outside the 8
middle incision at the 7
inner just inside the 6

Smaller OZ (5.5 mm to 7.5 mm) → 0.50 D to 1.00 D more

opposite that of the blade's direction as well as to maintain a proper perpendicular plane between the blade's footplates and the corneal surface. The Thornton ring also helps to maintain adequate intraocular pressure during placement of each incision.

Using the nomogram, the operative plan is established prior to surgery, carefully drawn out, and brought into the OR at the time of surgery and taped to the wall where it can be easily seen by the surgeon. This may seem elementary, but maintaining proper orientation and preventing any mix-ups in surgery are important considerations.

Thus prepared, the predetermined degrees of arc are carefully noted from the corneal marker and the blade positioned at either end of the planned incision (the triple edged arcuate diamond blade cuts either way) and then pressed into the cornea at the predetermined optical zone and slowly moved, on this optical zone, the full length of the planned incision. Care must be taken to keep the footplates perpendicular to the corneal surface. The incision is made slowly on a relatively dry cornea in order to best detect an early microperforation.

As the blade is advanced, a slow rotational movement of the handle between thumb and forefinger allows the narrow square-tipped blade to scribe a gentle arc along the curve of the marker at the given optical zone. Once completed, the incision is inspected and gently irrigated if necessary.

Summary

Using the instruments and nomograms now available, astigmatic keratotomy has been shown to be a reliable, safe and effective means of reducing pre-existing and surgically induced astigmatism.

Chapter 5

Reduction of Preoperative and Postoperative Astigmatism for Cataract Surgeons

R. Bruce Grene, MD
Richard L. Lindstrom, MD

Astigmatism and the Cataract Surgeon

Historical Development

The earliest application of astigmatic keratotomy was for a patient with unacceptable astigmatism following cataract surgery. In 1885, Schiotz, a Norwegian ophthalmologist, reported the case history of a 33-year-old patient who developed 19.5 diopters of astigmatism following cataract surgery.[1,2] Since that time, two trends characterize surgeons' efforts to control astigmatism: (1) corneal surgery, termed astigmatic keratotomy or AK, and (2) limbal surgery techniques addressing wound architecture and closure.

For the most part, AK has developed outside the mainstream of cataract surgery through the efforts of radial keratotomy specialists. Its recent integration into cataract surgery practice is a new development in the quest to achieve emmetropia for patients. Faced with the common complication of high astigmatism from long ICCE and ECCE incisions, cataract surgeons have developed various forms of incision architecture and wound closure to reduce astigmatism. Jaffe and Clayman's extensive review of 1,557 cataract cases compared eight suture techniques and four suture materials with thorough vector analysis of residual and induced astigmatism. Although mention is made of Troutman's limbal wedge resection technique,[3] no reference is made to astigmatic keratotomy. Nonetheless, their paper does foreshadow the integration of AK into cataract surgery by noting the ineffectiveness of wound compression as a means of controlling astigmatism. "Moreover, there is a decided tendency for the cornea to resume its preoperative curvature over long periods of time. This is more emphatic with postoperative wound compression than wound gape."[4] The recognition that limbal techniques were limited to wound recession and that wound compression was ineffective opened the door for the integration of AK into cataract surgery. The period from 1974 to 1994 shows mind-boggling progress in surgical technique to reduce astigmatism. Jaffe and Clayman don't mention wound length as a variable, showing a full 160° incision (Figure 5-1).[5] Today, only two decades later, surgeons can utilize a 3.5-mm incision which is astigmatically neutral. From this stage they can opt for either a corneal technique (AK) or a limbal technique (wound recession) to decrease pre-existing astigmatism.

Modern Significance of Astigmatism Reduction

The clinical significance of this dramatic evolution in astigmatism control lies in our ability to move from "not making patients worse" (through creating high postoperative astigmatism) to actually making them *better* than they were before surgery (by reducing pre-existing astigmatism). In addition, today's techniques afford much earlier visual rehabilitation and greater long term refractive stability. As we look ahead to the near future, today's techniques of astigmatism reduction will become increasingly important. *Multifocal intraocular lenses will demand emmetropia* to allow patients the full refractive benefits of these implants.

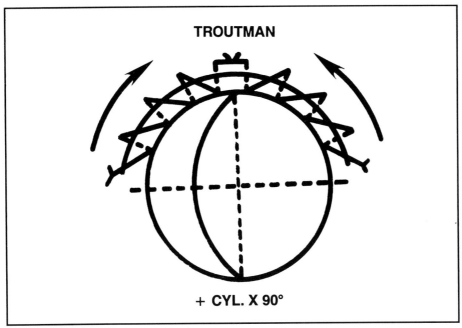

Figure 5-1. Shown is the Troutman continuous suture.

Modern Concepts

In 1974, surgeons struggled to avoid 4 D or more postoperative corneal astigmatism. As our ability to avoid extreme levels of postoperative astigmatism has advanced, we are challenged to detect more subtle and complex forms of astigmatism. Three forms of astigmatism impact patients' vision: regular, macroirregular and microirregular.

Regular corneal astigmatism remains the main concern for cataract surgeons. Regular astigmatism is a vector having both a magnitude (D) and direction (axis). Its direction is grouped into three categories; with-the-rule, against-the-rule, and oblique. Three diagnostic tests define regular astigmatism: refraction (refractive astigmatism), keratometry and computed topography (corneal astigmatism).

Macroirregular astigmatism[6,7] refers to irregular regional variations in corneal curvature and is best diagnosed with computed topography. Two clinical examples illustrate the importance of macroirregular astigmatism to cataract surgeons. Prior to cataract surgery, keratoconus shows inferotemporal steepening (Figure 5-2). Efforts to modify these patients' regular astigmatism are highly unpredictable and should be approached cautiously. Another clinical manifestation of macroirregular astigmatism is seen in the

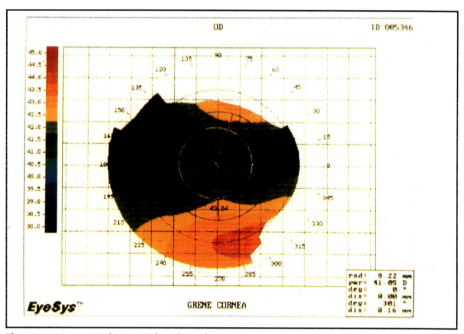

Figure 5-2. A topographic map of moderate keratotoconus.

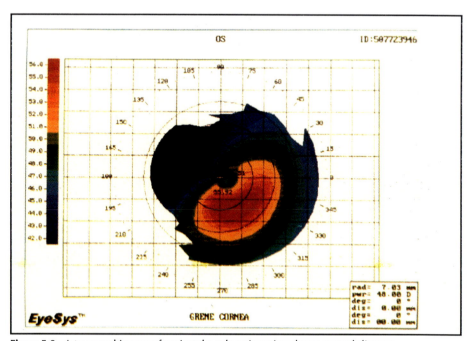

Figure 5-3. A topographic map of against-the-rule astigmatism due to wound slippage.

case of a slipped wound following long incision cataract surgery (Figure 5-3). This form of against-the-rule astigmatism is more difficult to manage with AK than symmetrical "bow tie" astigmatism. The surgeon should consider wound revision as an alternative to AK.

The third form of astigmatism, microirregular, is a major element in refractive surgery but less critical in cataract surgery.[8] With microirregular astigmatism, the keratometric mires appear distorted and the patient's refraction exhibits exaggerated hyperopia and astigmatism.[7] Failure to identify irregular astigmatism may lead to incorrect strategy for regular astigmatism reduction due to inaccurate refractive data. Sources of microirregular astigmatism include SPK (Superficial Punctate Keratopathy), corneal surgery and corneal scarring.

The refractive cataract surgeon must consider manifest refraction, manual keratometry and computed topography as preoperative and postoperative aids to identify all three forms of astigmatism. Their quantification intraoperatively remains an important but elusive goal.

Correction of Pre-existing Astigmatism at the Time of Cataract Surgery

Indications

The correction of pre-existing regular corneal astigmatism requires that each surgeon define their own indications for intervention. The incidence of astigmatism by magnitude and axis has been estimated by Nordan.[9] Approximately 80% of patients have 1.50 D or less pre-existing refractive astigmatism which can be approached by using a small-incision phacoemulsification technique (4.00 mm or smaller incision). The remaining 20% are candidates for either AK or wound recession to reduce their greater than 1.50 D astigmatism.

Koch and Lindstrom offer more restrictive selection criteria. "We consider reducing pre-existing astigmatism in patients whose astigmatism exceeds 2 D and whose fellow eye: (1) has 1.5 D or less of astigmatism, (2) has astigmatism at a different meridian than the operative eye, or (3) has a similar amount and meridian of astigmatism and is itself an imminent surgical candidate."[10]

Wound Manipulation

Surgeons can induce flattening of the steeper meridian by centering the cataract incision at this meridian and allowing wound slippage. By adopting a temporal surgical approach, when indicated, the surgeon can rely upon limbal wound manipulation for all cases and avoid the necessity of astigmatic keratotomy.

The technique of Koch and Lindstrom describes a fixed incision length and offers a nomogram for variable amounts of recession. *For a 6-mm incision, approximately 1 D of flattening can be assumed for each 0.25 mm of wound recession.* A maximum of 1 mm recession for 4 D effect is recommended.

Nordan utilizes a fixed amount of recession and utilizes variable incision lengths. A combined interrupted and running closure allows early cutting of selected interrupted sutures to titrate effect. A 6-mm wound is favored to negate 1.5 to 3.5 D cylinder. An 8-mm wound corrects 3.75 to 6 D cylinder.

Astigmatic Keratotomy

Astigmatic keratotomy for reduction of pre-existing astigmatism follows the basic guidelines of AK in conjunction with RK. One special consideration is the use of AK for with-the-rule and oblique cylinder. Maloney and Nordan favor wound revision over AK in these cases since the interaction of simultaneous limbal wound closure and keratotomy decrease the predictability of the effect of AK.[11] Another special consideration is the timing of the AK relative to cataract extraction. Shepherd, Nordan and Lindstrom perform AK prior to phacoemulsification. Maloney and Grene delay AK until the completion of phacoemulsification (Table 5-1).

Variables for Astigmatic Keratotomy

The five variables that determine the strength of astigmatic keratotomy are: (1) optical zone, (2) incision length, (3) incision depth, (4) incision number, and (5) configuration.

The smaller the optical zone, the greater the reduction in regular astigmatism and the greater the likelihood of inducing microirregular astigmatism. The most common choice of optical zone is 7 mm, representing the best balance of effect and side effects.

Incision length varies significantly from surgeon to surgeon. Those schools of approach utilizing multiple incisions generally call for shorter incision lengths, e.g. Maloney, 1.5 mm and 3.0 mm. In contrast, Grene and

Table 5-1.
Techniques of Five Surgeons

	For with the rule/oblique	For against the rule	Optical zone	Knife setting	Configuration	Incision lengths	Timing
Shepherd	AK	AK	7mm	90%	T	1mm/D	prior to phaco
Maloney	AK (poor results)	AK	7mm, 8mm	60%	T	1.5mm, 3.0mm	after phaco
Nordan	wound manipulation	AK	7mm	100%	T	3.5mm, 4.5mm	prior to phaco
Lindstrom	wound manipulation	AK	7mm	100%	Arc	30°, 45°, 60°, 90° arcs	after phaco
Grene	wound manipulation	AK	7mm	100%	T	3.5mm, 4.5mm	after phaco

Nordan use only three strengths of AK and longer incisions of 3.5 mm and 4.5 mm. Shephard's nomogram calls for 1 mm incision length per diopter of cylinder. Lindstrom's arcuate technique offers the greatest range of incision length: 30°, 45°, 60°, and 90°. Incision depth is somewhat less critical for AK than for RK. A vertical push blade technique generally creates 90% achieved depth when set at 100% (zero bias) of the pachymetry value at the intended operative location.

The number of incisions used for AK is balanced against incision length. Three potential options of equal strength include: (1) a single long incision, (2) two moderate length incisions 180° apart or (3) two short pairs of incisions 180° apart (Figure 5-4). Incision configuration is of relatively less importance than other variables. A recent comparison of 100 cases of arcuate keratotomy versus 100 cases straight transverse keratotomy by one of us (RBG) showed no statistically significant difference in outcome.

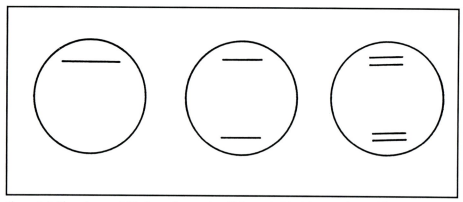

Figure 5-4. Three forms of AK of equal strength utilizing varied incision number and length.

Correction of Astigmatism After Cataract Extraction

The surgical reduction of astigmatism following cataract surgery varies in several important ways from techniques utilized at the time of cataract extraction. *Wound revision should be reserved for those cases with excessive astigmatism* (≥ 6 D) and slit lamp and computed topography evidence of wound slippage. Cases of low and moderate astigmatism are best addressed with AK. This applies to with-the-rule, oblique, and the more common against-the-rule forms. Nordan suggests modifying nomograms created for congenital astigmatism by multiplying the refractive cylinder by 70 percent. The resulting number should be used as the "working cylinder" to determine the strength of AK required. This reflects the greater effect of AK in postcataract patients (excluding those originally performed with astigmatically neutral incisions of 4 mm or less).

If AK is to be performed at the conclusion of phacoemulsification cataract extraction, the surgeon must pressurize the globe prior to performing the AK. In addition, it is valuable to mark the steep meridian and the center of the pupil prior to dilation and anesthesia. In other respects, AK can be approached as follows for congenital astigmatism.

ARC-T Technique of Astigmatic Keratotomy

In an effort to better understand astigmatic keratotomy, a group of nine surgeons performed arcuate transverse keratotomy on 159 eyes. Objectives included the determination of the effect of arcuate, transverse incisions on corneal and refractive astigmatism. The study assesses the reliability of postoperative manual keratometry by comparision to calcuated values. The predictability of the surgical nomogram is evaluated in the ARC-T Study (see Durrie/Schumer nomogram in Appendix I). Finally, complications and side effects associated with astigmatic keratotomy are reported.[12,13,14] The ARC-T Study represents the largest prospective, multicenter analysis of astigmatic keratotomy. For this reason, the ARC-T technique will be presented in detail below as a more detailed example of AK.

The patient is centered under the operating microscope. A bean-bag neck support is used to position the head (Vac Pack #11). The eye is anesthetized with topical anesthetic (proparacaine 0.5%). The center of the pupil is marked with a visual axis marker (Grene Katena #K3-8101). Center of pupil is marked with Grene Katena .60 mm at 7 mm if pachymetry is not available.

The corneal thickness is measured at the estimated steep meridian at approximately 7 mm using an ultrasonic pachymeter (DGH pachette). A front cutting blade (100 micron, 45°, Chiron Ophthalmics) is set under a micrometer microscope at 100% of the thinnest pachymetry measurement.

A solid blade lid speculum (Lester-Burch Katena #K1-5620) is inserted. Additional topical anesthetic drops are applied, followed by a drop of Celluvisc. Utilizing the Mendez degree gauge (Katena #K3-7900) and an arcuate incision marker (Grene Katena #K3-8101 or Lindstrom Katena #K3-7996), the incision guide marks are placed. The patient is directed to look nasally to bring a temporal incision to the center, inferior to bring a superior incision to the center, superior to bring an inferior incision to the center, or temporally to bring a nasal incision to the center. Secondary fixation is achieved using a fixation forceps (Bores Katena #K5-3250) at the limbus. The incision is carefully traced with a front cutting motion. The incision direction could be either clockwise or counterclockwise according to surgeon preference. The surface of the eye is irrigated with BSS in a 3 cc syringe witha 27-gauge cannula.

Postoperatively, each patient is placed on topical antibiotic and Celluvisc four times a day for one week. Anaprox DS (550mg) as needed for discomfort, and one Halcion (0.25 mg) for sleep are prescribed. Subsequent examinations are performed at two and four weeks. Exams include assessment of both near and distance vision, with and without correction. Manual keratometry, refraction, intraocular pressures, slit lamp evaluation, and in most cases, computed topography are performed.

In the ARC-T study, results for both refractive and keratometric change were analyzed with vector analysis. The Hollady, Cravy, Koch (H-C-K) method of vector analysis was selected for this presentation.[15]

Summary

Twenty years ago the most skilled anterior segment surgeons reported techniques for dealing with the then inevitable excessive astigmatism following 160° incision cataract surgery (Table 5-2). Today it is difficult to imagine 6, 8, and even 12 D induced astigmatism eight weeks after cataract surgery. This evolution (revolution!) has followed two convergent paths. The first path has been that of cataract surgeons whose relentless efforts have resulted in less invasive cataract incisions. Today we approach the reality of truly self sealing, astigmatically neutral 3-mm incisions. The other path has been that of refractive surgeons whose efforts in radial keratotomy have brought us the concepts and instrumentation vital to contemporary astigmatic keratotomy. The patient benefits from the integration of these paths into modern refractive cataract surgery. As we move forward to our goal of immediate, stable, multifocal emmetropia, it is important that surgeons and patients alike pause to recognize how remarkable is the miracle of modern cataract surgery.

Table 5-2.
Effect of Cutting Troutman Suture

Postoperative K	Weeks
-12.00 X 180°	9
-4.00 X 180°	10
-10.75 X 5°	7
-9.00 X 20°	7
-6.00 X 160°	12
-6.00 X 180°	11
-8.00 X 180°	6

References

1. Schiotz HA: in Fall von hochgradigem Hornhautastigmatismus nach Staarextraction. Besserung auf operativem Wege. *Archiv fur Augenheilkunde.* 1885;15:178-181.

2. Lindstrom RL: Lans distinguished refractive surgery lecture: the surgical correction of astigmatism: a clinician's perspective. *Refractive & Corneal Surgery.* Nov/Dec 1990; Vol 6:441-454.

3. Jaffe NS, Clayman HM: The pathophysicology of corneal astigmatism after cataract extraction. *Trans Am Acad Ophthalmol Otolaryngol.* 79 Jul/Aug OP-630, 1975.

4. Jaffe NS, Clayman HM: The pathophysicology of corneal astigmatism after cataract extraction. *Trans Am Acad Ophthalmol Otolaryngol.* 79 Jul/Aug OP-628-OP-630, 1975.

5. Jaffe NS, Clayman HM: The pathophysicology of corneal astigmatism after cataract extraction. *Trans Am Acad Ophthalmol Otolaryngol.* 79 Jul/Aug OP-616, 1975.

6. Grene RB, Lindstrom RL: Astigmatic keratotomy in the refractive patient: the ARC-T study: in Gills JP, Thornton SP, Martin RG, Sanders DR, eds, *The Surgical Treatment of Astigmatism.* Thorofare, NJ, SLACK, Inc., 1994.

7. Nordan LT, Grene RB: The importance of corneal aspericity and irregular astigmatism in refractive surgery. *Refract Corneal Surg.* 1990 May-Jun;6(3);200-4.

8. Grene RB: Astigmatism Chapter. In: Roy FH, ed, *Ophthalmic Surgery: Approaches of the Masters.* Philadelphia, PA, Lee & Febiger, In press.

9. Nordan LT, Maxwell WA, Davison JA, eds, *The Surgical Rehabilitation of Vision.* New York, NY, Gower Medical Publishing, 1992;23.23-28.

10. Koch DD, Lindstrom RL: Controlling astigmatism in cataract surgery. Seminars in Ophthalmology. Dec 1992;Vol 7-4:224-233.

11. Maloney WF: Transverse astigmatic keratotomy: an integral part of small incision cataract surgery. *J Cataract Refract Surg.* 1992 Mar;18:190-194.

12. Grene RB, Kenyon KR, Durrie DS, Lindstrom RL, Price FW, Whitson WE, Bodner BI, Binder PS, Gelender H: Astigmatism Reduction Clinical Trial: a multi-center prospective evaluation of the surgical results of arcuate keratotomy for the reduction of astigmatism, 1993. Submitted.

13. Price WP, Grene RB, Marks RG: Astigmatism Reduction Clinical Trial: one month & six month data with analysis of the results of two-stage astigmatic/myopic surgery versus one-stage surgery. Submitted.

14. Price WP, Grene RB, Marks RG: Astigmatism Reduction Clinical Trial: a multi-center evaluation of the predictability of arcuate keratotomy. Evaluation of surgical nomogram predictability. Submitted.

15. Holladay JT, Cravy TV, Koch DD: Calculating the surgically induced refractive change following ocular surgery. *J Cataract Refract Surg.* 1992;18:429-443.

Chapter 6

Arcuate Keratotomy
The Method, Technique and Instrumentation

Daniel S. Durrie, MD
D. James Schumer, MD

History

H. Schiotz was the first to report on an incisional procedure to correct astigmatism in 1885. L. Lans, in 1898, performed the first investigation of astigmatic keratotomy and formulated a description of the principles involved. In the 1940s, T. Sato established the principles of transverse keratotomy to correct astigmatism. S. Fyodorov in the 1970s developed numerous techniques to correct astigmatism while modernizing incisional refractive procedures. In the United States numerous clinicians, including Thornton, Nordan, Lindstrom, and Buzzard have refined incisional procedures for astigmatism. The ARC-T (Arcuate Transverse Keratotomy for the Reduction of Astigmatism) study which is a multicentered prospective evaluation has been completed with follow up data currently being collected and reported. The ARC-T study which shows good results with different surgeons using the same nomogram, will have the strongest appeal to the average refractive surgeon or cataract surgeon performing simultaneous astigmatic keratotomy.

Methodology

Prior to any type of refractive surgery, the surgeon is compelled to gather as much information as possible regarding the refractive state of the patient. A thorough dialog must take place between the patient and the surgeon. The surgeon must know the individual visual needs of the patient, while the patient needs to understand the realistic benefits and risks in order to give proper informed consent. Because the goal of refractive surgery is to decrease a patient's dependency on optical aids, monovision should be discussed with every patient regardless of age.

A refractive worksheet with all the necessary patient data should be used to facilitate completeness and ease of use. Figure 6-1 is an example of a refractive worksheet. Key features include age, dominant eye, uncorrected and best corrected vision, manifest refraction, spherical equivalent and keratometry. A schematic is available for the surgical plan.

Astigmatism is measured via the subjective refraction, keratometry and corneal topography. All are important to review prior to astigmatic keratotomy. These studies provide three distinct ways of confirming the magnitude and axis of the astigmatism and thereby confirming the surgical plan. If the data is conflicting, an explanation must be elicited.

Case 1

This 48-year-old male has recently failed on toric soft contact lenses.

Refraction: -3.00 - 3.50 x 70 = 20/20 3.25 - 3.00 x 83 = 20/25
Keratometry: OD 43.75 44.25 x 140 OS 43.25 44.75 x 147
Topography: No more than 1.50 diopters of astigmatism in the central cornea.

After the measurements were repeated and confirmed, a diagnosis of lenticular astigmatism was made. The retinoscopic reflex confirmed this diagnosis by providing the same measurement as the refraction. This demonstrates how a complete examination of the eye along with a thorough review of the measurements is crucial to obtaining a complete understanding of the refractive state of the patient. All of the existing data must confirm the

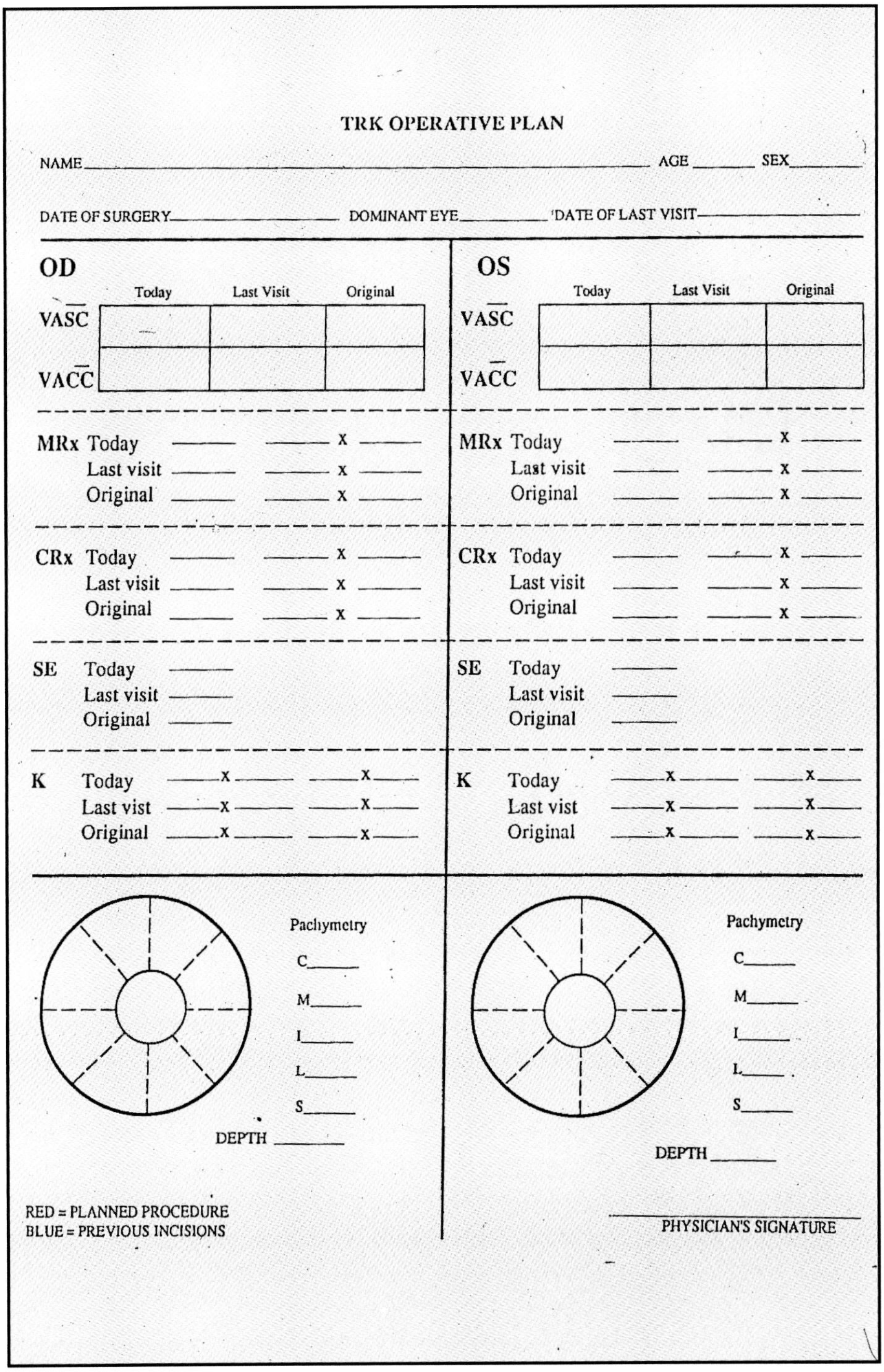

TRK OPERATIVE PLAN

NAME_____ AGE _____ SEX_____

DATE OF SURGERY_____ DOMINANT EYE_____ DATE OF LAST VISIT_____

OD

	Today	Last Visit	Original
VASC			
VACC			

MRx Today _____ _____ x _____
Last visit _____ _____ x _____
Original _____ _____ x _____

CRx Today _____ _____ x _____
Last visit _____ _____ x _____
Original _____ _____ x _____

SE Today _____
Last visit _____
Original _____

K Today ____x____ ____x____
Last vist ____x____ ____x____
Original ____x____ ____x____

Pachymetry
C_____
M_____
I_____
L_____
S_____

DEPTH _____

OS

	Today	Last Visit	Original
VASC			
VACC			

MRx Today _____ _____ x _____
Last visit _____ _____ x _____
Original _____ _____ x _____

CRx Today _____ _____ x _____
Last visit _____ _____ x _____
Original _____ _____ x _____

SE Today _____
Last visit _____
Original _____

K Today ____x____ ____x____
Last vist ____x____ ____x____
Original ____x____ ____x____

Pachymetry
C_____
M_____
I_____
L_____
S_____

DEPTH _____

RED = PLANNED PROCEDURE
BLUE = PREVIOUS INCISIONS

PHYSICIAN'S SIGNATURE

Figure 6-1. Refractive surgery worksheet.

patients refractive state before an operative plan can be considered. In this case corneal astigmatism was induced in order to compensate for the lenticular astigmatism.

Coupling

Coupling is the term given to the effect astigmatic keratotomy has on the overall curvature of the cornea. As astigmatic keratotomy flattens the steepest axis where the incision is made, it in turn steepens the flatter axis 90° away. In practical terms, this translates to astigmatic keratotomy correcting the cylinder while conserving the spherical equivalent. Gauss' Law describes that for a flexible and extensible surface, a bend in one meridian will be compensated 90° away in order to conserve the total curvature of the surface. As a balloon is squeezed, it flattens between your hands but steepens 90° away to conserve the total curvature. This concept translates well to the cornea and astigmatic keratotomy. Numerous studies have measured this effect for astigmatic keratotomy.[1,2,3,4]

Astigmatic keratotomy can be performed with either a curved or straight incision. Both provide a change in corneal curvature but their effect differs. A straight incision is measured in millimeters and has less effect when compared to a curved incision subtending the same angle. A curved incision maintains an equal distance from the optical center of the cornea throughout the incision (Figure 6-2). Because the corneal thickness increases from center to periphery, at any given optical zone the thickness is fairly constant. This is why a curved astigmatic incision has a uniform relative depth in the cornea (Figure 6-3). A straight incision, however, varies from the optical center (Figure 6-4). Therefore, the center of the incision, being closer to the optical center, is relatively deeper than the ends of the incision (Figure 6-5). A straight incision must be longer and actually subtend a larger angle in order have the effect of a curved incision.

Proper instrumentation in performing astigmatic keratotomy is essential for consistent predictable results. The ideal AK incision is a uniform 80% to 85% deep on the steep meridian(s). Ultrasound pachymetry is the first necessary step at the time of surgery. There are many variations of how to perform pachymetry prior to AK. Whether the measurement is taken at the incision site or adjusted from a reading done elsewhere on the cornea, a consistent reproducible pattern must be adopted. Our experience has produced excellent results by using only one blade depth setting for both astigmatic keratotomy and American technique radial keratotomy. The paracentral pachymetry readings (record the depth measured in each

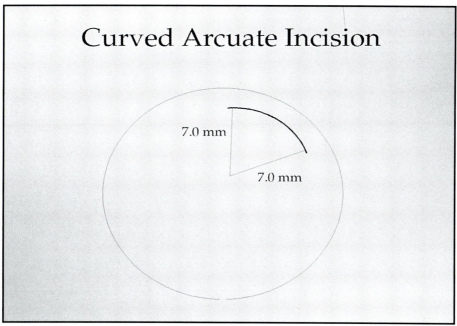

Figure 6-2. Depiction of a curved astigmatic keratotomy incision keeping equal distance from the optical center of the cornea.

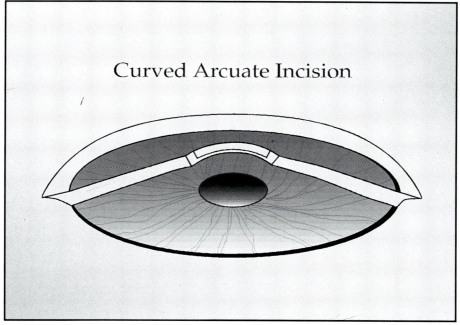

Figure 6-3. The relative depth of a curved astigmatic keratotomy incision maintains equal relative depth throughout the incision.

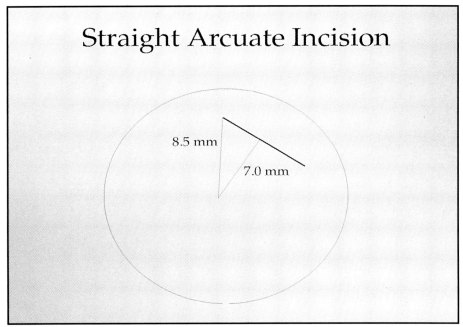

Figure 6-4. A depiction of a straight arcuate keratotomy incision showing the varying distance from the optical center along the length of the incision.

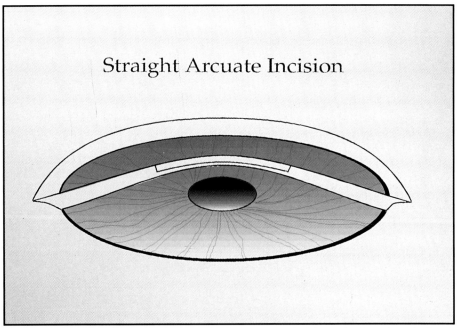

Figure 6-5. The relative depth of a straight astigmatic keratotomy incision varies throughout the length of the incision.

quadrant 3 mm from the center) are recorded and the blade is set at 110% of the thinnest of these measurements. This provides a conservative blade setting for both RK and AK, as well as, avoiding confusion over differing blade lengths depending on the quadrant or optical zone size. Setting the blade at 110% of the paracentral (3 mm) reading is similar to setting the blade at 100% of the 7-mm optical zone reading because the cornea becomes thicker as you move peripherally. This provides consistent 80% to 85% astigmatic keratotomy incision depths at the 7-mm optical zone. We do not see micro or macroperforations with this technique but the potential risk will always be present.

The actual depth obtained from a corneal incision performed with a diamond blade is dependent on several variables; blade length, blade design and technique of incision. A diamond blade will cut shallower than its length on the first pass of an incision. Also, the depth is shallower at the beginning of the incision than at the middle or end. The ratio of incision depth to blade length will vary with the blade design. A trifaceted blade cuts deeper than a back cutting blade which cuts deeper than a front cutting blade (Figure 6-6). Surgeon variables, such as the amount of pressure exerted and whether one

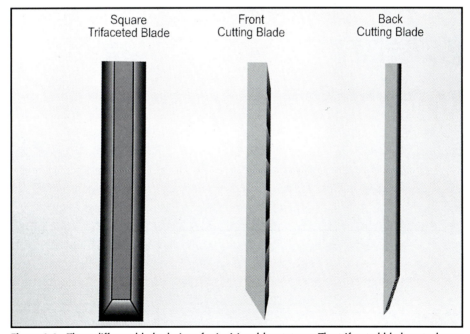

Figure 6-6. Three different blade designs for incisional keratotomy. The trifaceted blade cuts deeper than the front cutting blade which cuts deeper than a back cutting blade.

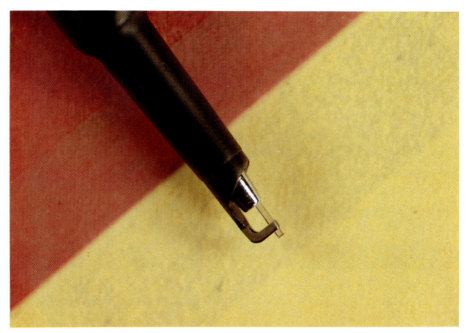

Figure 6-7. Photograph of the Chiron ARC-T trifaceted 150 micron blade.

pass or two are performed, also determine incision depth. It is crucial that as many of these variables as possible be kept constant. If changes in technique are planned, it is recommended to vary only one thing at a time, in order to avoid compounded errors and confusion over their origin.

The technique described has had excellent results. A trifaceted 150 micron blade, such as, Chiron's ARC-T blade is recommended for several reasons (Figure 6-7). The position of the blade forward in the support skis allows for excellent visibility during surgery. Because the blade is square, a light tap on the cornea leaves a small impression which can reassure the surgeon of the starting point of the incision. As a curved arcuate incision is performed, a trifaceted blade acts like a rudder in the tissue. The blade simply needs a gentle rotation in the finger tips in order to produce a curved incision. In addition, a square blade produces a more uniform incision with less feathering at the start of an incision. For enhancements, a square blade is easier to seat into a previous incision and less likely to produce a second or doubled incision.

The potential drawback to trifaceted blades is their ability to cut deeper if the blade is not held perpendicular to the cornea. Because the blade is square,

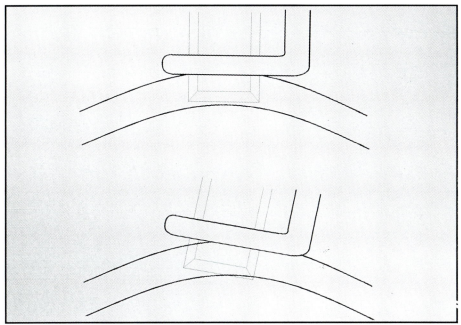

Figure 6-8. Trifaceted blade cutting at 80 to 85% depth when held perpendicular to the corneal surface may enter the anterior chamber if the perpendicular position is not maintained.

a tilt of the instrument away from perpendicular may cause a perforation as the 90° angle of the blade moves deeper into corneal tissue (Figure 6-8). Regardless of the blade design or technique, every refractive corneal incision needs a slow deliberate approach. The surgeon must be on constant guard for an aqueous leak which will prevent a microperforation from becoming a macroperforation.

The ARC-T (Astigmatic Reduction Clinical Trial) nomogram has the backing of a multicentered clinical trial in which we participated. The incisions are made at the 7-mm optical zone over a preplaced corneal marker. The markers vary in degrees; 30°, 60° or 90° (Figure 6-9). The placement of the marker is guided by a hand held ring with markings that determine the axis (Figure 6-10). The twelve o'clock position on the limbus can be marked prior to the procedure in order to facilitate proper orientation.

The ARC-T nomogram varies the length and number of incisions at a 7-mm optical zone according to the age of the patient and magnitude of astigmatism (Figure 6-11). It is important to realize this nomogram is for congenital astigmatism. Large variations in response may be attained if the astigmatism is postsurgical (cataract or penetrating keratoplasty), pterygium

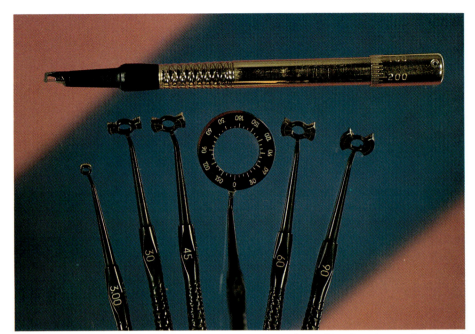

Figure 6-9. Photograph of the arcuate keratotomy instruments for marking the axis as well as the 30°, 60° and 90° markers.

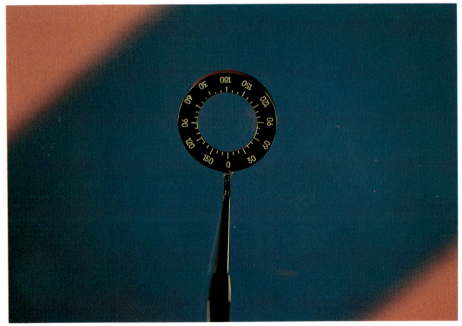

Figure 6-10. The axis marker for the arcuate keratotomy instrument set.

ASTIGMATISM REDUCTION CLINICAL TRIAL

EXPLANATION FOR USE OF NOMOGRAM

- Identify patient's age and the diopters of refractive cylinder that you wish to correct.

- Find the patient's age in the first column on the left.

- Move to the right until you've reached the surgery result closest to the refractive cylinder of the patient. In order to avoid overcorrection, it is suggested that you select a surgical goal somewhat less than the actual refractive cylinder. The column heading tells you which surgery is needed to achieve this result.

EXAMPLE

45-year-old patient with a refractive cylinder of 3.75

- 3.75 falls between 2.60 and 3.90

- A single 90° ARC-T or a paired 45° ARC-T will correct 2.60 diopters of cylinder

- A paired 60° ARC-T will correct 3.90 diopters of cylinder

- The recommendation in this case is to do a paired 45° or a single 90° ARC-T

EXPECTED SURGICAL RESULTS WERE CALCULATED USING LINDSTROM'S FORMULA

$$\Delta D = [100 + (AGE - 30) \times 2] \times [\Delta D \text{ at age } 30] \times 0.01$$

Figure 6-11A. The arcuate keratotomy nomogram.

	Surgical option				
	2 X 30°		2 X 45°		
AGE	1 X 45°	1 X 60°	1 X 90°	2 X 60°	2 X 90°
20	0.80	1.20	1.60	2.40	3.20
21	0.82	1.23	1.64	2.46	3.28
22	0.84	1.26	1.68	2.52	3.36
23	0.86	1.29	1.72	2.58	3.44
24	0.88	1.32	1.76	2.64	3.52
25	0.90	1.35	1.80	2.70	3.60
26	0.92	1.38	1.84	2.76	3.68
27	0.94	1.41	1.88	2.82	3.76
28	0.96	1.44	1.92	2.88	3.84
29	0.98	1.47	1.96	2.94	3.92
30	1.00	1.50	2.00	3.00	4.00
31	1.02	1.53	2.04	3.06	4.08
32	1.04	1.56	2.08	3.12	4.16
33	1.06	1.59	2.12	3.18	4.24
34	1.08	1.62	2.16	3.24	4.32
35	1.10	1.65	2.20	3.30	4.40
36	1.12	1.68	2.24	3.36	4.48
37	1.14	1.71	2.28	3.42	4.56
38	1.16	1.74	2.32	3.48	4.64
39	1.18	1.77	2.36	3.54	4.72
40	1.20	1.80	2.40	3.60	4.80
41	1.22	1.83	2.44	3.66	4.88
42	1.24	1.86	2.48	3.72	4.96
43	1.26	1.89	2.52	3.78	5.04
44	1.28	1.92	2.56	3.84	5.12
45	1.30	1.95	2.60	3.90	5.20
46	1.32	1.98	2.64	3.96	5.28
47	1.34	2.01	2.68	4.02	5.36
48	1.36	2.04	2.72	4.08	5.44
49	1.38	2.07	2.76	4.14	5.52
50	1.40	2.10	2.80	4.20	5.60
51	1.42	2.13	2.84	4.26	5.68
52	1.44	2.16	2.88	4.32	5.76
53	1.46	2.19	2.92	4.38	5.84
54	1.48	2.22	2.96	4.44	5.92
55	1.50	2.25	3.00	4.50	6.00
56	1.52	2.28	3.04	4.56	6.08
57	1.54	2.31	3.08	4.62	6.16
58	1.56	2.34	3.12	4.68	6.24
59	1.58	2.37	3.16	4.74	6.32
60	1.60	2.40	3.20	4.80	6.40
61	1.62	2.43	3.24	4.86	6.48
62	1.64	2.46	3.28	4.92	6.56
63	1.66	2.49	3.32	4.98	6.64
64	1.68	2.52	3.36	5.04	6.72
65	1.70	2.55	3.40	5.10	6.80
66	1.72	2.58	3.44	5.16	6.88
67	1.74	2.61	3.48	5.22	6.96
68	1.76	2.64	3.52	5.28	7.04
69	1.78	2.67	3.56	5.34	7.12
70	1.80	2.70	3.60	5.40	7.20
71	1.82	2.73	3.64	5.46	7.28
72	1.84	2.76	3.68	5.52	7.36
73	1.86	2.79	3.72	5.58	7.44
74	1.88	2.82	3.76	5.64	7.52
75	1.90	2.85	3.80	5.70	7.60
AGE	1 X 45°	1 X 60°	1 X 90°	2 X 60°	2 X 90°
	2 X 30°		2 X 45°		

Figure 6-11B. The arcuate keratotomy nomogram continued.

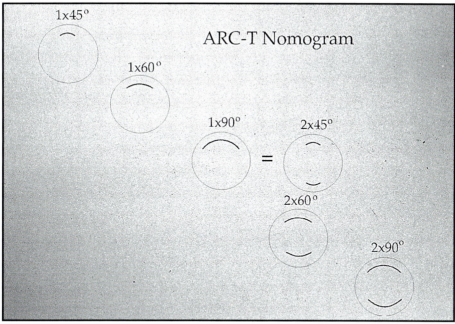

Figure 6-11C. The arcuate keratotomy nomogram continued.

induced or posttrauma. The forces present in these situations may lead to large responses. Therefore, extreme conservatism is prudent.

After the eye is anesthetized with Tetracaine or 4% Lidocaine, the patient is comfortably reclined. Constant communication with reassurance from the surgeon and staff promotes relaxation by instilling confidence in the patient. Systemic sedation, such as oral Valium, can facilitate a comfortable atmosphere for the patient but is usually not necessary. After the eye is prepped and draped, a lid speculum is placed. The patient is asked to fixate at a fixation light specifically designed for refractive procedures. The surgeon should be coaxial with the patient's fixation. This allows for the proper positioning to mark the optical center of the cornea by using the center of the patient's pupil. A 3-mm optical zone marker is recommended because it allows the surgeon a chance to check the position of the mark and make a second mark if necessary. If a mark is placed in the center of the pupil with the Sinsky hook, then fixation is disturbed for the patient and the surgeon cannot double check the centration.

Arcuate Keratotomy Combined with Cataract Extraction

Arcuate keratotomy performed at the time of cataract surgery has become a very successful approach to refining the refractive outcome for this procedure. There are several important considerations that need to be addressed with regard to combining AK with cataract extraction.

Before a cataract surgeon contemplates performing AK as an adjunct to cataract extraction, he/she must know how their current surgical technique affects astigmatism. We recommend that 95% (2 standard deviations) fall within + or - 0.50 D of a consistent shift in the cylinder. Depending on the surgical technique (extracapsular, scleral-tunnel phaco or clear-corneal phaco) and suture technique (nylon, mersilene or no-stitch), patients may need to be followed one year or longer until a "stable" cylinder is obtained. This could be obtained through a chart review as long as the surgical technique has remained constant.

Several differences in the AK technique described above will be necessary when performed at the time of cataract extraction. *Unless your cataract extraction technique is performed under topical anesthesia, the patient will not be able to fixate for location of the optical center of the cornea.* The anatomical center of the cornea should then be used by marking with a 5-mm optical zone marker. The appropriate ARC-T marker can then be used at the 7-mm optical zone.

The best time to perform AK during cataract surgery is currently up for debate, but we feel it should be before the anterior chamber is entered. Some surgeons like to begin their incision or tunnel in order to help insure that the case will proceed as planned, and then, before the anterior chamber is entered, perform the AK. Once the anterior chamber is entered and surgery progresses, hypotony and corneal swelling ensue which would affect the result of an incisional keratotomy. Because of the additional variables in combining AK with cataract extraction, a conservative approach to the ARC-T nomogram is strongly encouraged. This nomogram was developed for congenital astigmatism with no other variables considered. Please keep this in mind when using the nomogram outside of this criterion.

References

1. Lundergun MK, Rowsey JJ: Relaxing incisions: corneal topography. *Ophthalmology.* 1985; 92:1226-1236.

2. Merlin U: Curved keratotomy procedure for congenital astigmatism. *J Refract Surg.* 1987; 3:92-97.

3. Duffy RJ, Vivanti NJ, et al: Paired arcuate keratotomy: a surgical approach to mixed and myopic astigmatism. *Arch Ophthal.* 1988; 103:477-488.

4. Hofmann RF: The surgical correction of idiopathic astigmatism. N. Sanders DR, Hofmann RF, Ansalz JJ, eds, *Refractive Corneal Surgery.* Thorofare, NJ, SLACK, Inc., pp 241-290, 1986.

Chapter 7

Intraocular Correction of Refractive Errors

Harry B. Grabow, MD

Introduction

"WE, THE PEOPLE, ..." of the anterior segment ophthalmic surgery societies "... in order to form a more perfect union ..." of incident light rays and the refracting surfaces of the human eye, have entered the age of mass emmetropization of the population. Indeed, all of the technical subject matter in this text is dedicated toward that singular purpose. Historically, those of us who have chosen as our life's work to deal with human vision and its flaws have always held as the ideal, the "gold standard" (if you will), the state of emmetropia. It, therefore, has always been and continues to be our lifelong mission and commitment to produce clear, functional vision for those members of our society who were unfortunately born with, or who later developed, ametropia.

In the beginning, we might say that we were in the "spectacle age" of ametropia correction, as the idea of placing a lens on the eye or in the eye had not yet been conceived. However, even during this time, Tadini, in approximately 1709, is recorded as one of the first to suggest the concept of an artificial intraocular lens for aphakia, which at that time was generally the result of intentional or unintentional couching. Casamada, in 1790, is credited with the first attempt at intraocular lens implantation following intracapsular cataract removal. Unfortunately, with no method for fixation, this first IOL attempt was unsuccessful, as the heavy crystal pseudophakos was seen to disappear rapidly into the vitreous as "an idea before its time."

If we are to be complete in discussing the topic at hand, as denoted by the title of this chapter, we must not limit our thinking to intraocular lenses as the only method of correction or to aphakia as the only correctable refractive error. Other intraocular methods have been proposed and tried besides the use of an "artiphakos." The idea of *clear lensectomy* for high myopia was first proposed as early as 1890 by Fukala but was not performed successfully until the latter half of the present century. Another ocular organelle, other than the lens, was considered modifiable for the correction of myopia by Sato in the 1930s. We are all familiar with his early attempts at perhaps the first keratorefractive procedure, *radial keratotomy*, performed from the endothelial side of the cornea which soon proved to be another failed effort at an intraocular technique to correct an ametropia ... another "idea before its time."

The concept of using implantable devices with refractive power to correct ametropia is not new to us, but was an idea reborn in our time with the first successful intraocular lens implanted by Harold Ridley in England, in 1949, to correct surgical aphakia. Within a few short years, the mid-1950s, Ridley's European colleagues had already begun to apply the new concept to include phakic errors of refraction. Stampelli, Danheim, Barraquer and Choyce implanted the first intraocular lenses for the correction of myopia. However, as we have observed with previous technological developments, these early lenses were doomed to fail, only to be relegated, for the next two-to-three decades, to the fate, once again, of an "idea before its time."

These early phakic intraocular lenses failed due to our lack of knowledge of the proper design requirements and safe implantation techniques. Lens manufacturing in the 1950s was crude and primitive by today's standards. Lenses were thick, heavy, and not sized to the spaces that were to receive them. The consequences of corneal endothelial and crystalline lenticular trauma were previously not known, but rapidly became apparent.

The concept of the intraocular correction of ametropias with the seductive possibility of man-made emmetropia remained in the back of our minds but was tabled for a couple of decades while we concentrated our efforts first at perfecting spherical IOLs for the correction of aphakia. The proper design requirements for the successful long-term retention of these intraocular prostheses were finally determined, as well as five different locations, methods of fixation, materials, and methods for safe implantation, not the least of which include viscoelastics, capsulorhexis, phacoemulsification, foldable lenses, sutureless small-incision technology and topical anesthesia. This concept of surgical emmetropia continues to drive our technological machine and has led us now, in the light of the success we have had with the spherical correction of aphakia, to return our efforts to the intraocular correction of the phakic ametropias ... now as an "idea whose time has come!"

Toric IOLs

Astigmatism is an optical phenomenon resulting from the aberrant alteration of parallel rays of light passing through non-spherical refractive media of the eye, namely the cornea and the lens. The aberrant focal separation of light rays, in the case of regular, symmetrical, orthogonal astigmatism, results in the optical creation of the well-known conoid of Sturm, thereby "converting an otherwise normal monofocal eye into a multi-focal eye."[1]

Much has been said in earlier chapters in this text about incisional techniques, particularly the various forms of cataract incision and astigmatic keratotomy, designed to alter the topographic anatomy of the cornea. Additionally, excisional techniques, such as the special ablation patterns used with excimer keratectomy, are also currently being actively studied worldwide to modify and reshape the cornea in order to neutralize refractive astigmatism.

However, as the development of phakic refractive IOLs is presently limited, as were aphakic IOLs initially, to spherical models for the phakic correction of hyperopia and myopia, the first IOL for the correction of astigmatism has also appeared as a combined model for the simultaneous correction of aphakia. Phakic toric IOLs (i.e., IOLs for the simultaneous correction of phakic myopia + astigmatism or hyperopia + astigmatism) have yet to be manufactured. These are next on our list and, I predict, will be seen in our surgical lifetime.

The manufacturing of toric IOLs is not difficult and certainly could have occurred at the outset of modern IOL production in the 1970s; however, we—as an industry of ophthalmic surgeons—were not ready for them. At that time we could not make our incision for a rigid PMMA IOL for correction of aphakia that was consistently and predictably astigmatically neutral. It is obvious that incisional astigmatic neutrality is a prerequisite to using a toric IOL. Not until phacoemulsification was combined with astigmatically neutral IOL incisions could we begin to conceive of approaching the concept of aphakic toric IOLs.

Preliminary Studies

Several retrospective and prospective demographic and surgical analyses were conducted in the United States around 1990 under the direction of Donald R. Sanders (University of Illinois). The first study was designed to assess how much astigmatism is actually present in our patient cataract population. Are its prevalence and severity significant enough to warrant corrective measures, particularly the costly development of an aphakic toric IOL? Two sets of data were available for retrospective analysis; those of Robert G. Martin (Southern Pines, NC) and of myself. In Martin's series of 596 eyes, 23% were found to have presented with 1.5 or more diopters of keratometric cylinder preoperatively (Figure 7-1). My series of 1,235 eyes showed 18% with 1.5 or more diopters of keratometric cylinder (Figure 7-2).

A theoretical computer model was then designed by Sanders, using vector analysis, to determine how far off-axis an aphakic toric IOL could rotate postoperatively before it would lose its beneficial effect and actually add to the pre-existing refractive cylinder. He found that such an IOL could rotate up to 30° off-axis (one clock-hour) before it, theoretically, would lose its astigmatism neutralizing effect and begin to add toric power.

A preliminary prospective clinical study was then undertaken by John R. Shepherd (Las Vegas, NV) and myself to study the rotational stability of the STAAR 4203 one-piece plate-haptic 10.5 mm silicone foldable IOL (Figure 7-3) when placed in the intact capsular bag through an intact capsulorhexis. In a combined group of over 50 eyes, 91% of these lenses were observed to be positionally stable, rotating less than 15° postoperatively (Figure 7-4).

These preliminary studies set the stage for the subsequent United States FDA clinical trial of the STAAR 4203T, the first one-piece foldable silicone aphakic toric IOL.

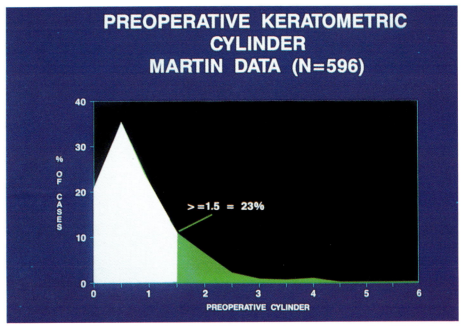

Figure 7-1. Naturally occurring astigmatism (1.5 D or greater) in cataract extraction (RG Martin and DR Sanders).

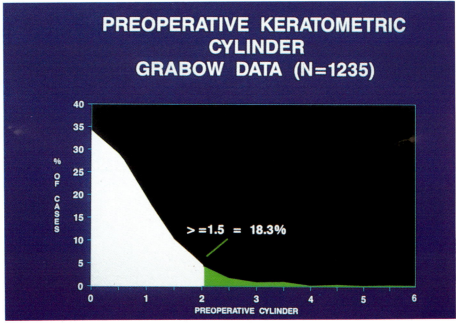

Figure 7-2. Naturally occurring astigmatism (1.5 D or greater) in cataract population (HB Grabow and DR Sanders).

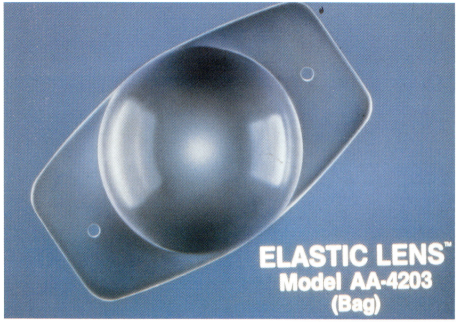

Figure 7-3. The STAAR AA-4203 one-piece plate-haptic foldable silicone spherical IOL.

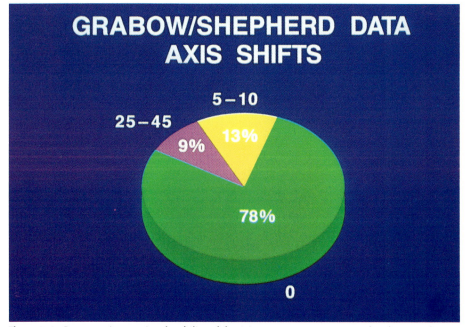

Figure 7-4. Postoperative rotational stability of the STAAR AA-4203 10.5 mm plate-haptic spherical IOL (DR Sanders).

Clinical Trials

The idea of using artificial lenticular astigmatism in the form of a toric pseudophacos is one that has historically emerged on two continents, Asia (Japan) and North America (United States). The first report of human sighted-eye cases of toric IOL implantation at the time of cataract extraction was presented at the San Diego meeting of the *American Society of Cataract and Refractive Surgery* (ASCRS) in April of 1992 by Kimiya Shimizu of Tokyo. The lens used in this initial study was a three-piece design with a 5.5 mm by 6.5 mm oval polymethylmethacrylate (PMMA) optic and 13.0 mm polypropylene modified-C loops manufactured by NIDEK. The oval optic had two holes to facilitate rotation, and the line between the holes corresponded to the axis of the toric correction in the IOL (Figure 7-5). This prototype model was manufactured in two toric powers, +2.00 and +3.00 diopters.

Two questions were of interest in this initial study. Firstly, what was the postoperative rotational stability of IOLs of this traditional posterior chamber design, obviously a critical factor in order to reduce and not induce refractive astigmatism and, secondly, to what degree do +2.00 and +3.00 D of

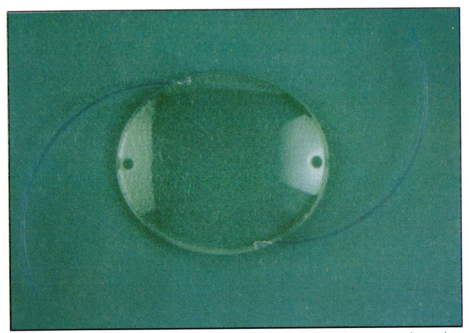

Figure 7-5. Three-piece PMMA toric-aphakic IOL with 5.5x6.5 mm and 13.0 mm polypropylene modified-C loops (K Shimizu, NIDEK).

pseudophakic toricity correct pre-existing keratometric cylinder as measured at the spectacle refractive plane? Shimizu found that this lens design permitted the IOL to stay within 20° of the axis of implantation in 70% of cases. In the remaining 30%, the lenses rotated off-axis more than 20° due to the effect of fibrotic contraction of the capsule on the haptics. In the eyes in which the IOL stayed on-axis, the lens with 2.00 D of cylinder corrected approximately 1.00 D of refractive cylinder, while the IOL with 3.00 D of cylinder corrected approximately 2.00 D of refractive astigmatism.

Shimizu is now studying a second design of toric IOL. This model is a one-piece, all-PMMA style with a 5.25 mm round optic and 12.5 mm modified-C loops (Figure 7-6). To date, he has published no data regarding the results of this lens. Shimizu has also had considerable experience with the rectangular design plate-haptic STAAR 4203 silicone IOL and feels that this design might be more resistant to the rotational effects of capsular fibrosis.

The American experience began in 1992 with the United States FDA clinical trial of the STAAR 4203T. This model is slightly different from its spherical predecessor (4203) in three ways. Firstly, the optic has a toric power of approximately +2.00 D on one surface which, if it is to produce its full

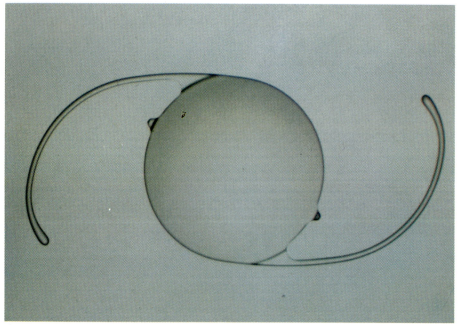

Figure 7-6. One-piece PMMA toric-aphakic IOL with 5.25 mm round optic and 12.5 mm modified-C loops (K Shimizu, NIDEK).

effect, is to be implanted anteriorly. Secondly, the periphery of the optic is scored with two small lines on the toric surface denoting the toric axis, which aligns also with the long axis of the haptics (Figure 7-7). Thirdly, the overall length of the 4203T is 10.8 mm, slightly longer than the 10.5 mm spherical 4203, to further insure rotational stability.

The STAAR toric study is presently in Phase I. It is a randomized prospective study of 125 toric cases and 125 controls. The minimum criterion for entry into the study is 1.00 D of preoperative, naturally occurring corneal astigmatism, as determined by keratometry. Eyes are excluded from this pilot study if they have corneal disease, glaucoma, uveitis, an axial length 24.00, or are an only eye.

Technique of STAAR 4203T Implantation

In order to avoid off-axis surgical placement of the toric IOL, the axis is marked before any block type of anesthesia is administered. The patient is seated at a slit lamp in which one ocular has been replaced with a reticle. The

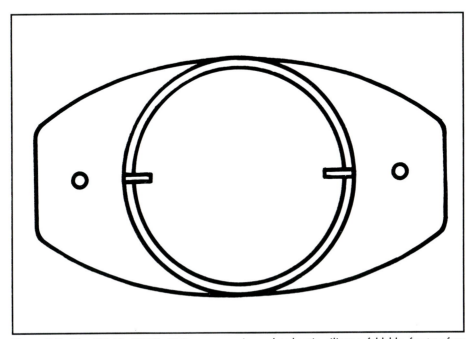

Figure 7-7. The STAAR 4203T, 10.8 mm one-piece plate-haptic silicone foldable front-surface toric-aphakic IOL.

axis of steep curvature is marked by placing a small dot on the limbal conjunctiva with a sterile gentian violet marking pen.

Cataract extraction is then performed by phacoemulsification through either a scleral or a corneal sutureless, self-sealing incision with an intact anterior capsulorhexis and intact posterior capsule. The 4203T is injected into the capsule in the same fashion as the 4203 in one step (Figure 7-8), using the MicroSTAAR Injector (Figure 7-9) and the 45° beveled cartridge (Figure 7-10), making sure to load the lens cartridge with the alignment marks anterior. After removal of the viscoelastic from the capsular bag (Figure 7-11) and the anterior chamber, the lens is rotated until the toric axis marks line up with the gentian violet marks at the limbus. The sutureless incision is closed by inflation of the anterior chamber with BSS through the side-port paracentesis incision.

Early Results

As of this writing, almost 125 STAAR 4203T foldable toric IOLs have been implanted in the United States study. Additional cases have been performed outside of the United States study in Europe. The purpose of the United States

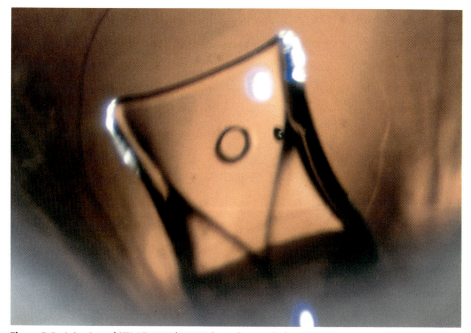

Figure 7-8. Injection of STAAR 4203/4203T through capsulorhexis.

study is two-fold: to determine the degree of rotational stability of the longer 10.8 mm design and the degree to which 2.00 D of front-surface toric power in the IOL actually corrects refractive cylinder at the spectacle plane.

Preliminary analysis of the first cases revealed that in 94%, the IOLs remained relatively stable, rotating less than 30°. In the group that remained within 5° of implantation axis (88%), an average reduction of 1.3 D of

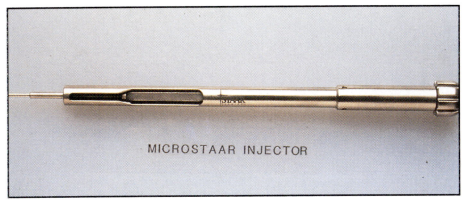

Figure 7-9. MicroSTAAR injector for one-step injection of STAAR foldable silicone IOLs.

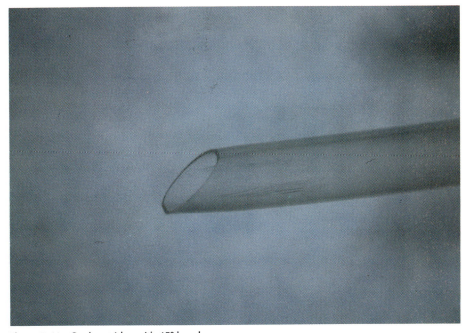

Figure 7-10. Oval cartridge with 45° bevel.

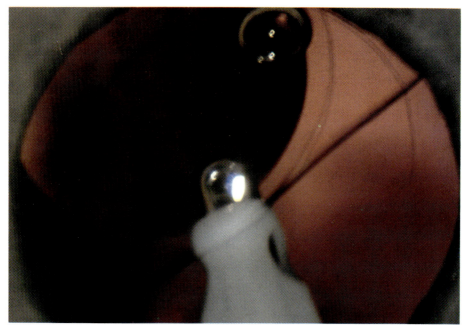

Figure 7-11. Automated removal of viscoelastic from behind the IOL in the capsular bag.

refractive cylinder was corrected. In the group in which the lens rotated between 5° and 15° (30%), an average reduction of 1.2 D of refractive cylinder was seen. In one case that rotated 40° off-axis, 0.4 D of refractive cylinder was added to the preoperative amount which, in itself, is less astigmatism than the average of many cases by incisional induction. In the best-case analysis of 20/40 or better corrected visual acuity, the toric and control groups demonstrated no statistically significant difference.

The preliminary conclusions of the study to date are that aphakic toric implantation is not only safe but is also predictable at reducing existing corneal-refractive astigmatism. An apparent average of about 65% of the keratorefractive cylinder is corrected with an equal amount of cylinder correction in the IOL, a ratio of 2.0 to 1.3 in this study. Conversely, if custom aphakic toric IOLs are to be manufactured in the future, one might assume that the IOL may require about 35% more toric power than the corneal-refractive cylinder to achieve, postoperatively, an eye with a spherical refraction. In actuality, a fixed linear relationship between corneal and implant toricity may not exist, but rather a nomogram may need to be developed following future clinical trials at correcting high degrees of corneal cylinder, especially in combination with phakic high myopia.

Future Advantages

Once fully developed, it is possible that toric correction in both cataract replacement IOLs and phakic refractive IOLs may become the standard of practice of many surgeons. Toric IOLs are *more predictable* than keratorefractive procedures and are also *reversible*, while keratorefractive procedures are not. In addition, they are more cost-effective than laser keratorefractive procedures, less painful, produce immediate results, and have almost no surgeon learning curve.

Phakic IOLs

Of the current world population of over 5.2 billion people, it has been estimated that approximately 800 million are "myopes," and that 63 million of these live in the United States. It has been further estimated that 95% of myopes (760 million) are between -1.00 and -6.00; and, conversely, that 5% (40 million) are "high" myopes, greater than -6.00.

Surgery for ametropia, as we have discussed, has naturally involved attempts at altering the two refractive areas of the eye, the cornea and the lens. Corneal refractive surgery has involved incisions, excisions, heat, cold, onlays, inlays, blades, lathes, and laser beams. The major advantage to choosing to modulate the cornea is that, most of the time, the procedure remains a closed-eye technique, avoiding the risks and complications of open-eye procedures. Disadvantages of the various keratorefractive procedures have included limited predictability, lack of reversibility, delayed onset of desired effect, lack of long-term stability, corneal de-stabilization, optical zone cicatrization, postoperative pain, glare, cost inefficiency, and undeveloped surgical proficiency.

Lenticular refractive surgery, on the other hand, has involved lensectomy, with or without a replacement IOL, and now phakic IOL implantation. The obvious advantages of *lenticulo*refractive surgery include precise predictability,[2] reversibility, immediate onset of desired effect, long-term stability, little or no adverse effect on corneal stabilization or optical zone clarity, little or no postoperative pain, cost efficiency, and an already familiar surgical procedure. The disadvantages of lenticular surgery, as mentioned, include all of the well-known risks and complications of open-eye procedures as well as, in the particular case of prepresbyopic clear lensectomy, loss of the vital function of accommodation.

The remaining content of this chapter will be devoted to phakic IOL implantation. This may be the only intraocular surgical refractive procedure with the potential for accuracy, immediacy, predictability, reproducibility, reversibility, and a future level of safety that may, not only equal the results of keratorefractive procedures, but might exceed them without altering intraocular anatomy or physiology (including accommodation). What follows is a brief overview of some of the work that has been done to date by some of our contemporary colleagues in our quest to conquer ametropia.

Anterior Chamber Lenses

I begin here, the anterior chamber, not only because it is the first location for implantation anatomically encountered upon opening the eye, but it is also the first site of phakic implantation attempted historically. It all began in Europe in the 1950s, a few short years after Ridley had performed the first successful implant for aphakia across the English Channel in 1949. Strampelli and Danheim were the first to try rigid PMMA anterior chamber IOLs for myopia, soon to be followed by Choyce and Barraquer. Barraquer was the first to report a long-term study of a large series, a five-year follow-up on 239 cases. In this first series, many lenses had to be removed due to corneal decompensation or (what later came to be called) "UGH" syndrome, uveitis-glaucoma-hyphema.

Except for two cases performed in 1969 in Russia by Svyatoslav Fyodorov, there was about a twenty-five year hiatus in phakic refractive lens implantation, while the technology of manufacturing and implanting IOLs for aphakia continued to develop. Phakic myopic IOL implantation of the anterior chamber was re-inaugurated in 1986 with the more modern lens design of Georges Baikoff of Marseille, France. Baikoff chose the successful four-point fixation design of Kelman because of its successful track record as an angle-supported anterior-chamber IOL for aphakia. Almost simultaneously, in May of 1987, Akira Momose of Japan developed and implanted his first glass-optic, two-piece polyamide-looped phakic myopic anterior chamber lens (ACL). Donald Praeger, formerly of West Palm Beach, Florida, was a proponent of the concept and collaborator with Dr. Momose, and he was the first surgeon to report the results of these lenses. Subsequent implantations of the one-piece Baikoff lens were undertaken in 1989 by Thomas Neuhann of Munich, Germany, and in 1990 by Roberto Zaldivar in Mendoza, Argentina, Peter Choyce in England, and by Al Neumann in Florida, who was the first United States surgeon to implant the Momose lens. In 1991, the first United States FDA-approved study of a phakic anterior-chamber IOL for myopia was begun by Herb Kaufman in New Orleans. Thus, the renewed interest and activity in the intraocular correction of ametropia by "modern" phakic anterior-chamber implantation was resumed with vigor on four continents: Europe, Asia, North America and South America.

Baikoff Lens

This one-piece PMMA anterior-chamber IOL is a four-point fixation lens modeled after the successful Kelman design and is manufactured currently by DOMILENS in Lyon, France. The first design implanted by Dr. Baikoff in 1986, model ZB, had a 4.5 mm optic with steep shoulders and a 25° vault angle. The lens was implanted through a sutured temporal incision under viscoelastic protection. The refractive results were good, with 80% of eyes achieving ± 1.00 D of emmetropia. However, by 1989, only three years later, 10% of cases were demonstrating progressive endothelial cell loss and some actually demonstrated areas of endothelial cell absence due to IOL touch with eye rubbing.

The design of the lens was subsequently changed to the currently implanted model ZB5MF (Figure 7-12). This design has a smaller optic of 4.0 mm with a 0.5 mm "carrier ring" making the total optic diameter 5.0 mm. The shoulders are flatter than previous models and the vault angle is 5° shallower at 20° (Figure 7-13). The lens is manufactured in three sizes, 12.5, 13.0 and 13.5 mm, and is recommended to be fit using the traditional external measurement of the horizontal corneal diameter, "white-to-white," plus 1.0 mm. It is also recommended that the preoperative endothelial cell count be 2500 cells/mm^2 or greater and that the anterior chamber depth be a minimum of 3.2 mm for IOL powers of -7.00 to -15.00 and 3.4 mm for -16.00 to -20.00. This model of Baikoff IOL can be used for myopia ranging from -7.00 to -24.00. The manufacturer (DOMILENS) presently provides guidelines for choosing IOL powers (Table 7-1).

Baikoff ACL Procedure

This ACL implantation technique is really no different from any ACL implantation technique, for those of us familiar with primary or secondary

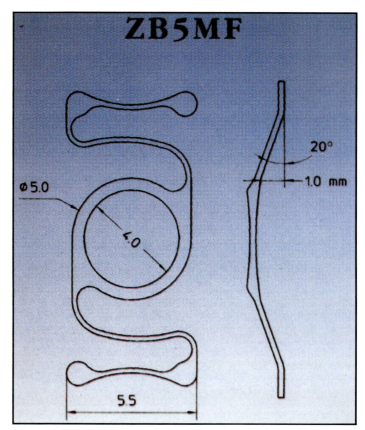

Figure 7-12. Baikoff phakic AC-IOL for myopia (DOMI- LENS, Lyon, France).

aphakic ACL procedures. The pupil is rendered miotic preoperatively and intraoperatively, as needed. A 6.0 mm temporal clear-corneal incision is made and the IOL is advanced until the leading haptic rests in the nasal angle and the trailing haptic is tucked into the temporal angle without iris tucking as indicated by pupillary distortion. A patent iridotomy should then be performed. The viscoelastic is removed and the incision is sutured. Operative gonioscopy is performed to verify haptic locations.

Baikoff Lens Results

Although Dr. Baikoff, himself, has selectively implanted over 150 of his design lenses since 1986, the combined world experience to-date is estimated to be over 3,000 eyes. The current model ZB5MF (Figure 7-14) is now in a five-year multi-center study in France. Early results of cases with a minimum of 18 months of follow-up are encouraging with regard to IOL power

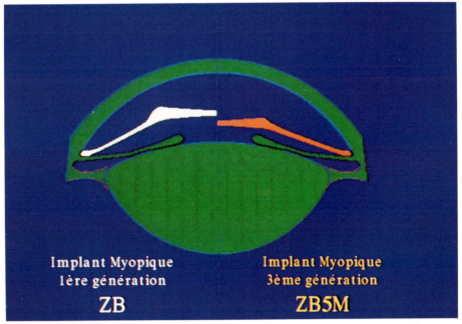

Implant Myopique
1ère génération
ZB

Implant Myopique
3ème génération
ZB5M

Figure 7-13. Baikoff phakic AC-IOL for myopia. Schema compares 1st and 3rd generation designs.

calculation predictability, demonstrating 75% within 1.00 D of the expected refractive result. Considering the wide range of myopia in the series, -7.00 to -24.00, averaging -12.20, and lack of previous studies on which to base IOL power calculation nomograms, these early refractive results are excellent. So far, only three eyes have required IOL exchange for incorrect power, which is remarkable with current A-scan technology, especially since many of these eyes have axial lengths over 28.00 mm.

From a technical aspect, three cases were observed by Saragoussi and co-workers[3] to develop the classic postoperative signs of anterior chamber IOLs that are too long for the space intended: deformed pupils, iris tucking, chronic low-grade inflammation, posterior synechiae and sector iris atrophy.

Although this is a very small number of cases of oversizing, the fact that this phenomenon is present at all is indicative that accurate sizing of modern anterior chamber IOLs remains a technical problem to be dealt with. Another phenomenon well known to be associated with anterior chamber IOLs is pupillary block with iris bombé and secondary angle closure, an alteration of the anterior segment internal milieu referred to as "internal iris prolapse" by Peter Choyce in the 1970s. Four such eyes with phakic Baikoff IOLs have required laser iridotomy postoperatively, indicating that these lenses, not unlike their aphakic predecessors, necessitate an iridectomy or iridotomy at the time of implantation.

A few cases of the earlier model ZB Baikoff ACL with steep shoulders and a vault angle of 25° were reported to have a cell loss after 12 months as high as 53%[4] and actual acellular areas due to IOL edge touch.[5] The current-generation ZB5MF Baikoff ACL, with flatter shoulders and a shallower vault angle of 20°, is demonstrating much lower cell loss, averaging 4.9% ± 5.8 at

Table 7-1.

IOL Power Guideline (DOMILENS)

REF	IOL
- 8.00 to -10.00	Same
-11.00 to -15.00	Same + 1.00
-16.00 to -20.00	Same + 2.00
Over -20.00	Max -18.00

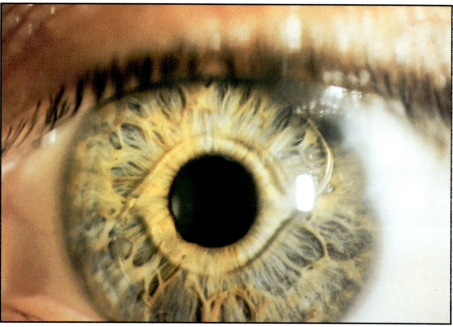

Figure 7-14. Baikoff ZB5MF phakic AC-IOL in-situ.

the 18-month report.[6] Although no data have yet been officially published in the very limited 5-case United States FDA study directed by Kaufman, in a "Letter to the Editor," by Dr. Kaufman in June 1992, he stated, ". . . our five patients have absolutely no endothelial cell loss, no inflammation, and no apparent adverse anatomical changes."[7]

One of our major concerns with intraocular surgery on high myopes has always been the possibility of postoperative retinal detachment. The risk of this complication may be greater following clear lensectomy; however, our ability now to improve these eyes without disturbing the lenticular and posterior segment architecture may render refractive lensectomy obsolete. So far, only three cases of retinal detachment following phakic implantation of the anterior chamber have been reported.[8] These three eyes all received ZB5M IOLs in 1991 and, despite appropriate preoperative evaluation, developed rhegmatogenous detachments six weeks, eight months, and ten months postoperatively. Surgical reattachment was successful in all cases resulting in best-corrected visual acuity of 20/100 in two cases and 20/400 in the third case after secondary vitrectomy and membrane peeling for proliferative vitreoretinopathy.

All surgeons performing phakic refractive implantation of highly myopic eyes routinely include peripheral retinal examination and prophylactic treatment of pathology in their preoperative protocol. It is unknown whether or not the three cases reported above were destined to have spontaneous detachments even without their implant surgery, as all three eyes had axial lengths greater than 28.90 mm. It is certainly a credit to these and to the technology investigators that so few detachments have been reported, considering that over 3,000 procedures have been performed in eyes already at high risk.

This French study under the direction of Baikoff is presently on-going, as is the American study directed by Kaufman. The final five-year data are yet to be obtained. Whether further design modifications in this IOL will be necessary is, as yet, unknown.

Momose "Spider" Lens

This two-piece ACL, designed and first implanted in 1987 by Akira Momose, has a haptic design that resembles the configuration of a spider (Figure 7-15). The optic is made of glass with an index of refraction of 1.62 and is held in a circular polyimide ring from which the four curved haptics originate. The vault angle of this lens, only 6°, is much shallower than the 20°

of the second-generation Baikoff lens. The overall lengths available were from 12.5 mm to 13.5 mm and were implanted, like the Baikoff lenses, using the external horizontal corneal diameter plus 1.0 mm.

These lenses were implanted in a prospectively designed study, as reported by Praeger, Momose and Muroff[9] in 23 eyes from May 1987 to November 1988. The AC depth, as measured by ultrasonography in the accommodated state, was greater than 3.3 mm in all cases, and all eyes had a preoperative endothelial cell count greater than 2800 cells/mm². The range of myopia preoperatively was -8.00 to -20.25. Twelve eyes received -8.00 IOLs, six received -10.00 IOLs, and five received -13.00 IOLs.

Momose Lens Results

All eyes implanted with the Momose phakic ACL attained refractive stability by six weeks, presumably not as a result of any intraocular or IOL phenomenon, but rather as a result of wound healing. All of the eyes had residual myopia postoperatively ranging from -0.25 to -8.00, except for two eyes. These began -8.00 and -8.75 preoperatively, both received -8.00 IOLs, and both turned out to be overcorrected at +1.25 and +0.50, respectively.

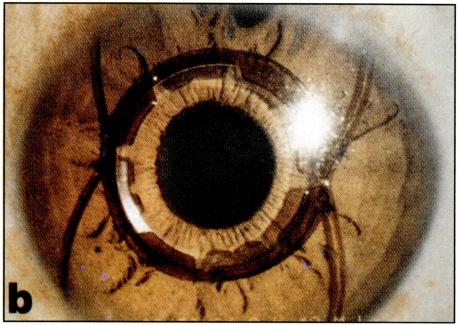

Figure 7-15. Momose "spider" phakic AC-IOL in-situ (courtesy of Albert Neumann, MD).

Two other eyes, one -14.25 and the other -17.50, had also received -8.00 lenses, apparently empirically at the start of the study, and these resulted in gross undercorrections of -8.00 postoperatively. All the rest stabilized in the -2.00 to -6.00 range, some of the more highly myopic undercorrected eyes (near -20.00), demonstrating a need for an IOL power greater than -13.00.

None of these 23 eyes lost any lines of visual acuity. In fact, one of the impressive benefits observed was an actual improvement in *corrected* visual acuity of one to three lines in 13 of the eyes (56%) postimplantation. This phenomenon may be explained by the increased magnification provided by the IOL.

Surgically, this small series of cases demonstrated no operative or postoperative complications. The endothelial cell loss one year postoperatively averaged 5.3% and remained stable with this model of IOL out to two and three years.

Albert Neumann of Deland, Florida, has recently reported on three cases of Momose lenses (AAT Enterprises, Thiells, NY) implanted since 1990. His brief report noted the postoperative formation of peripheral anterior synechiae (PAS) around the polyimide loops in the angle; however, this did not seem to be of any immediate clinical significance. In addition, he reported an endothelial cell loss of 7% with these three cases, not significantly different from that reported by Praeger, et al, in Dr. Momose's cases.

No further reports of this myopic ACL have been observed by this author and it is unknown whether these lenses are still being manufactured or implanted.

Iris-Fixated Lenses

This IOL fixation location is not new but may be unfamiliar to the young American implant surgeon. In fact, over 40,000 Worst iris-claw lenses have been implanted for aphakia since 1978, a good percentage of which were performed by Dr. Daljit Singh in Armitsar, India. Like the angle-supported anterior chamber lenses, these iris-supported IOLs are also not dependent on the lens or lens capsule for fixation and, therefore, for aphakia, are not limited in their use by the method of crystalline lens removal, intracapsular or extracapsular. The use of this lens design in the phakic eye is also not new and actually antedates the 1986 resumption date for all other modern styles of phakic IOL. Jan Worst, of the Netherlands, implanted his first iris-claw IOL in a phakic eye in 1980 to produce pupillary occlusion in a patient with otherwise intractable diplopia. The first Worst iris-claw lens actually implanted to correct myopia was performed in November 1986 in Germany by Paul Fechner.

Worst "Iris-Claw" Lens

This lens, designed by Jan Worst, is manufactured by OPHTEC in Groningen, Holland. It is a one-piece design (Figure 7-16) of PERSPEX CQ-UV PMMA, available in powers from -5.00 to -20.00 in 1.0 D steps. A detailed nomogram has been worked out by G. L. van der Heijde using anterior chamber depth and keratometry, as well as refraction (Table 7-2). The optic diameter is 5.0 mm with an overall haptic diameter of 8.5 mm. The vault height is 0.9 mm and, by schematic cross-sectional analysis (Figure 7-17), is represented to have significantly greater distance from the corneal endothelium than its angle-supported cousin. Its lobster claw-like split haptics are designed to fixate by incarceration of a knuckle of the mid-peripheral anterior iris stroma (Figure 7-18), intended to allow the pupil to fully dilate and constrict without IOL interference (Figure 7-19).

Worst "Iris-Claw" Procedure

As with phakic anterior chamber lens implantation, the pupil is constricted preoperatively and intraoperatively, as needed, for protection of the crystalline lens from operative trauma and to provide the substrate to which this ICL is to be attached. A superior limbal incision is made measuring approximately 7.0 mm and two side-port paracenteses at the three and nine o'clock meridians. Viscoelastic is instilled and a Sheets glide may be used. The IOL is placed in position with special holding forceps and a knuckle of iris is brought into each haptic claw mechanism using a special hook through the adjacent paracentesis. The incision is sutured following peripheral iridotomy and the viscoelastic is removed. Oral and topical steroids are administered postoperatively, as well as mydriatics.

Worst "Iris-Claw" Results

Fechner and co-workers in Germany had the largest initial experience with the Worst iris-claw myopia lens. In 1993, they reported the five-year results of 127 eyes implanted between November 1986 and November 1991.[10] In this series, 68% of eyes came to within 1.00 D of the desired postoperative refraction. Although there were no operative complications, 7% of eyes had

Specifications

Material	:	Perspex CQ-UV PMMA
Construction	:	Single Piece PMMA
Power Availablity	:	-5.0 to -20.0 dpt
		(1.0 dpt steps)
Optic	:	Convex-Concave
Optic Diameter	:	5.0 mm
Overall Diameter	:	8.5 mm
Total Height	:	0.9 mm
Weight	:	10 mg in air (-15 dpt lens)
Sterilization	:	Ethylene Oxide (ETO)
Fixation	:	To mid-peripheral iris stroma

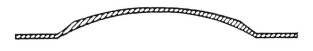

Section at -5.0 Diopter

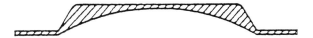

Section at -25.0 Diopter

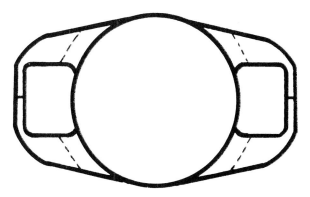

Figure 7-16. Worst "iris-claw" phakic IOL for myopia.

Table 7-2.

van der Heijde Nomogram

AC :	—	2.5 mm	—	—	3.0 mm	—	—	3.5 mm	—	—	4.0 mm	—
K :	38	43	48	38	43	48	38	43	48	38	43	48

Specs												
-1	-1.2	-1.2	-1.3	-1.3	-1.3	-1.3	-1.3	-1.3	-1.4	-1.3	-1.4	-1.4
-2	-2.3	-2.4	-2.4	-2.4	-2.5	-2.5	-2.5	-2.5	-2.6	-2.5	-2.6	-2.7
-3	-3.4	-3.5	-3.5	-3.5	-3.6	-3.7	-3.6	-3.7	-3.8	-3.7	-3.9	-4.0
-4	-4.5	-4.6	-4.6	-4.6	-4.7	-4.8	-4.7	-4.9	-5.0	-4.9	-5.0	-5.2
-5	-5.5	-5.6	-5.7	-5.7	-5.8	-5.9	-5.8	-6.0	-6.2	-6.0	-6.2	-6.4
-6	-6.5	-6.6	-6.8	-6.7	-6.8	-7.0	-6.9	-7.1	-7.3	-7.1	-7.3	-7.6
-7	-7.5	-7.6	-7.8	-7.7	-7.9	-8.1	-7.9	-8.1	-8.4	-8.1	-8.4	-8.7
-8	-8.4	-8.6	-8.8	-8.7	-8.9	-9.1	-8.9	-9.2	-9.4	-9.2	-9.5	-9.8
-9	-9.3	-9.5	-9.7	-9.6	-9.8	-10.1	-9.9	-10.2	-10.5	-10.1	-10.5	-10.9
-10	-10.2	-10.5	-10.7	-10.5	-10.8	-11.1	-10.8	-11.1	-11.5	-11.1	-11.5	-11.9
-11	-11.1	-11.4	-11.6	-11.4	-11.7	-12.0	-11.7	-12.1	-12.4	-12.1	-12.5	-12.9
-12	-12.0	-12.2	-12.5	-12.3	-12.6	-12.9	-12.6	-13.0	-13.4	-13.0	-13.4	-13.9
-13	-12.8	-13.1	-13.4	-13.2	-13.5	-13.8	-13.5	-13.9	-14.3	-13.9	-14.4	-14.9
-14	-13.6	-13.9	-14.2	-14.0	-14.4	-14.7	-14.4	-14.8	-15.2	-14.8	-15.3	-15.8
-15	-14.4	-14.7	-15.0	-14.8	-15.2	-15.6	-15.2	-15.7	-16.1	-15.6	-16.1	-16.7
-16	-15.2	-15.5	-15.9	-15.6	-16.0	-16.4	-16.0	-16.5	-17.0	-16.4	-17.0	-17.6
-17	-16.0	-16.3	-16.7	-16.4	-16.8	-17.2	-16.8	-17.3	-17.8	-17.2	-17.8	-18.5
-18	-16.7	-17.1	-17.4	-17.2	-17.6	-18.0	-17.6	-18.1	-18.6	-18.0	-18.7	-19.3
-19	-17.5	-17.8	-18.2	-17.9	-18.3	-18.8	-18.3	-18.9	-19.4	-18.8	-19.5	-20.1
-20	-18.2	-18.6	-18.9	-18.6	-19.1	-19.6	-19.1	-19.6	-20.2	-19.6	-20.2	-20.9
-21	-18.9	-19.3	-19.7	-19.3	-19.8	-20.3	-19.8	-20.4	-21.0	-20.3	-21.0	-21.7
-22	-19.6	-20.0	-20.4	-20.0	-20.5	-21.0	-20.5	-21.1	-21.7	-21.0	-21.7	-22.5
-23	-20.2	-20.7	-21.1	-20.7	-21.2	-21.8	-21.2	-21.8	-22.5	-21.7	-22.5	-23.2
-24	-20.9	-21.3	-21.8	-21.4	-21.9	-22.5	-21.9	-22.5	-23.2	-22.4	-23.2	-24.0
-25	-21.5	-22.0	-22.4	-22.0	-22.6	-23.1	-22.5	-23.2	-23.9	-23.1	-23.9	-24.7
-26	-22.2	-22.6	-23.1	-22.7	-23.2	-23.8	-23.2	-23.9	-24.6	-23.7	-24.5	-25.4
-27	-22.8	-23.3	-23.7	-23.3	-23.9	-24.5	-23.8	-24.5	-25.3	-24.4	-25.2	-26.1
-28	-23.4	-23.9	-24.4	-23.9	-24.5	-25.1	-24.5	-25.2	-25.9	-25.0	-25.9	-26.7
-29	-24.0	-24.5	-25.0	-24.5	-25.1	-25.7	-25.1	-25.8	-26.6	-25.6	-26.5	-27.4
-30	-24.6	-25.1	-25.6	-25.1	-25.7	-26.4	-25.7	-26.4	-27.2	-26.2	-27.1	-28.0

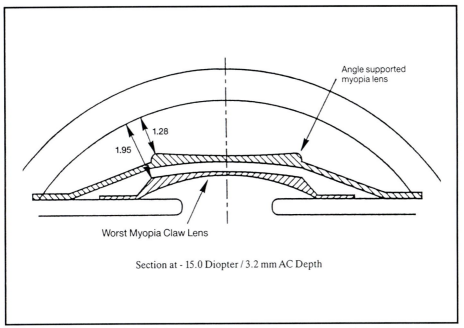

Figure 7-17. Worst "iris-claw" phakic myopic IOL schematic comparison with Baikoff AC-IOL.

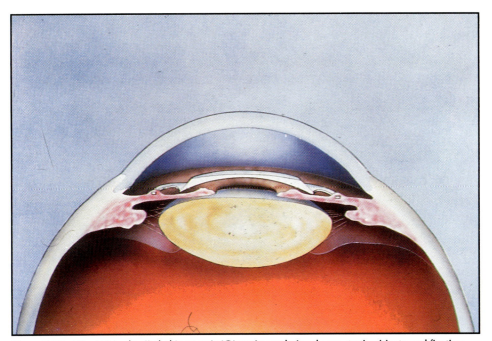

Figure 7-18. Worst "iris-claw" phakic myopic IOL: artist rendering demonstrating iris stromal fixation.

shown progressive endothelial cell loss. Fechner recommends that eyes to receive this lens have a minimum of 3.5 mm of anterior chamber depth and that they be followed with annual cell counts for the remainder of life. After this initial five-year study of the iris-supported phakic IOL, he suggested that the posterior chamber may be a safer location for the long-term retention of a phakic IOL.

Jose Menezo in Valencia, Spain, is also very experienced at using the iris-claw lens, having implanted the aphakic model for twelve years. From January 1990 to March 1993, he implanted 90 phakic myopic IOLs.[11] The average preoperative spherical equivalent in this series was -14.00. Postoperatively, the average spherical equivalent of the implanted group was -0.21. The percentage of uncorrected eyes able to see 20/30 or better, postoperatively, was 30%. Two lenses had to be removed; one had lost iris fixation and was intermittently in contact with the endothelium, and one was the incorrect power. Dr. Menezo also noticed progressive endothelial cell loss within the first year, averaging 3.3% at six months and 7.5% at one year. This particular report of April 1993 did not have the availability of cell count data beyond one year, so it is not yet known if the cell loss has continued or if it has stabilized.

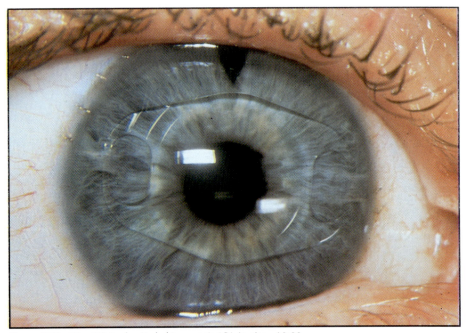

Figure 7-19. Worst "iris-claw" phakic myopic IOL in-situ, -18.00.

Later in the same year, in October 1993, OPHTEC (the Dutch company that manufactures the iris-claw lenses) in conjunction with CHIRON-INTRA OPTICS of the USA published an Interim Report of an on-going prospective study by surgeons in five countries: Annen in Switzerland, Budo and Termote in Belgium, Menezo in Spain, Sener in Turkey, and Worst in the Netherlands. The report is of 99 eyes in 67 patients implanted with lens powers from -6.00 to -20.00, with -12.00 being the most common power. At six months, 81% of eyes refracted between -1.00 and + 1.00 spherical equivalent. As reported by Praeger with the Momose spider lens, 52% of these iris-claw eyes improved from two to four lines in corrected visual acuity. So far, this group of eyes has lost an average of 7% of endothelial cells at the one-year count.

Some of the recent findings of the users of this lens have led to a minor controversy. Dr. Jorge Alió y Sanz of Spain reported chronic flare and cell in nine cases and stopped implanting this lens.[12] Dr. Worst took issue with the report of Dr. Alió, citing the results of the much larger series of Dr. Fechner, et al, in Germany.[13] This kind of open controversy is healthy and stimulating; however, only the findings of well-constructed and well-executed long-term prospective clinical trials will provide us all with the answers to our questions. At that time, the course of action of responsible investigators will be obvious.

Posterior Chamber Lenses

The posterior chamber is the aqueous filled space lined anteriorly by the posterior surface of the iris, peripherally by the ciliary sulcus, and posteriorly by the zonule and anterior lens capsule. This space is the first location in the eye to successfully be implanted with an artificial lens (Ridley 1949) for aphakia following extracapsular cataract extraction. As modern cataract surgery and aphakic implant technology evolved in the 1970s and 1980s, the intact evacuated lens capsule became the preferred location for PMMA IOL implantation, avoiding the mishaps of blind sulcus loop placement and chronic alteration of the blood-aqueous barrier. Lenses that were originally manufactured as long as 14.0 mm for sulcus placement were stuffed into the 10.5 mm collapsed capsule through can-opener capsulectomies. Thus, the first *capsular* IOLs were actually posterior chamber IOLs; and, hence, from that time on, all lens designs intended for implantation behind the iris, whether 12.5 mm PMMA for the sulcus or 10.5 mm silicone for the bag, were collectively and erroneously called "posterior chamber lenses."

In the same year (1986) that Baikoff in France and Fechner in Germany began phakic PMMA implant fixation in the anterior chamber angle and on the anterior iris surface, Fyodorov and Zuyev in Moscow began phakic silicone implantation of the posterior chamber.

Fyodorov Lens

The original first-generation Fyodorov phakic posterior chamber lens of 1986 resembled a "collar button." It was a one-piece silicone lens with a small 3.0 mm front-surface concave optic (Figure 7-20) that projected anteriorly through the pupil (Figure 7-21) and was fixated by a haptic in the posterior chamber (Figure 7-22). The small 3.0 mm size of this first-generation optic caused nocturnal edge glare and monocular diplopia and was replaced in 1990 with a second-generation design. This second model has a larger optic, measuring approximately 4.5 mm, set in a rectangular plate haptic (Figure 7-23) that is approximately 6.0 mm wide and of variable lengths. The design

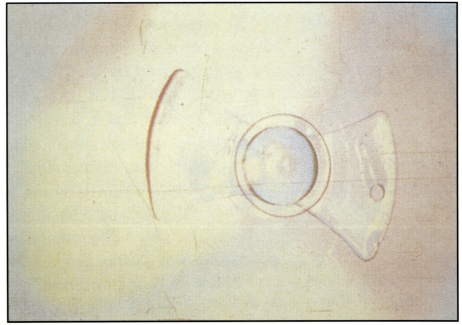

Figure 7-20. Fyodorov first-generation "collar-button" phakic myopic IOL.

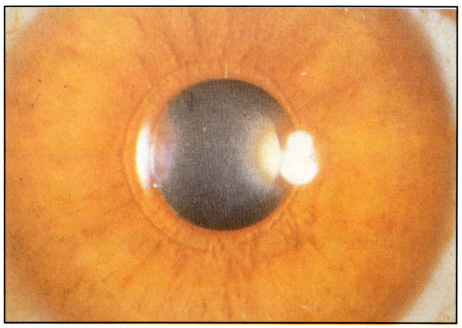

Figure 7-21. Fyodorov "collar-button" phakic myopic IOL in-situ.

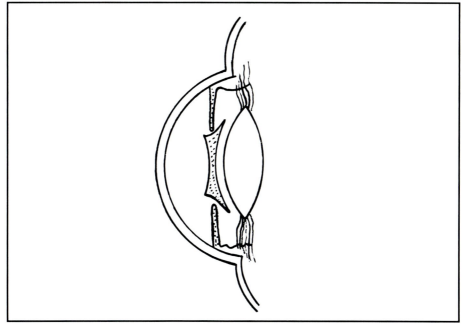

Figure 7-22. Fyodorov "collar-button" phakic myopic IOL-schema.

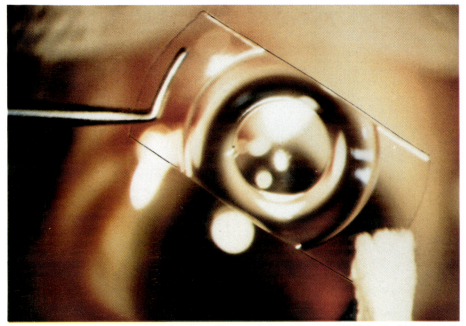

Figure 7-23. Fyodorov posterior-chamber silicone phakic IOL (ADATOMED GmbH, Munich, Germany; courtesy of P. Fechner, MD).

resembles the plate-haptic STAAR aphakic models in the United States, except that the optic is concave on its front surface and the plate haptic is concave on its back surface. This second-generation model is made of a different material, incorporating collagen into the silicone in order to make the material hydrophilic. Theoretically, this would make the IOL not only physically softer in aqueous but possibly less traumatic to endothelium and more bio-compatible for better long-term retention between its two adjacent mobile intraocular structures (iris and lens) (Figure 7-24).

Fyodorov Lens Procedure

Although this lens is of soft material, whether of silicone only or of silicone-collagen copolymer, a very few cases have been implanted in a folded, rolled, or injected fashion through a small incision, and those only began in the latter half of 1993. The Russian group, the Department of High Myopia Surgery, established by Fyodorov at his institute in Moscow headed by Viktor K. Zuyev, has the largest experience with phakic posterior chamber implantation, now over 1,000 cases.

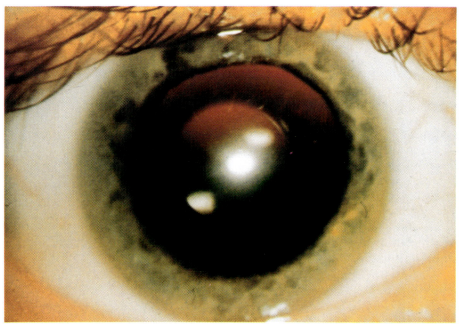

Figure 7-24. Fyodorov posterior-chamber silicone phakic IOL in-situ (ADATOMED GmbH, Munich, Germany; courtesy of P. Fechner, MD).

The method used by the Russian group involves a 6-7 mm superior limbal incision for flat (unfolded) implantation of the soft, delicate lens. Viscoelastic is used only when needed, as many cases can be performed under aqueous only. The leading haptic is slowly and gently fed through the incision and guided by gentle nudges through the dilated pupil, across the anterior lens capsule, and behind the inferior iris. The superior footplate is then placed into the superior posterior chamber by slight dialing with posterior pressure. The IOL may then be gently massaged, a maneuver designed to try to get the corners of the footplates to fixate between zonular fibers. The pupil may then be made miotic and iridotomy may be performed. The incision is then sutured.

In Russia, this procedure is reserved for myopia -8.00 and higher. The Russians have developed a nomogram to be used as a guide to selecting IOL power (Table 7-3). The procedure is usually performed in adults with myopia stable for at least one year. However, the Russians have also used their lens to treat congenital unilateral high myopia in children. Most of these cases are in patients over age 11 years. Posterior scleroplasty is performed first, using strips of dura apparently harvested from human cadavers. Following demon-

Table 7-3.

Fyodorov IOL Power Guide

REF	IOL
Up to -10.00	Same
-10.00 to-15.00	Same + 1.00
-15.00 to-20.00	Same + 2.00

stration of axial length stability for at least one year, the phakic myopic posterior chamber lens is implanted. The Russians have also developed a hyperopic model used for eyes +5.00 or greater.

Fyodorov Lens Results

The Russian group recently reported the results of 450 of the phakic first-generation "collar-button" posterior chamber IOLs (PCLs) that were implanted in patients 19 to 53 years of age with myopia from -10.00 to -23.00.[14] One of the first questions most observers of this procedure usually ask regards the rate of cataract formation. Remarkably, in this first series of phakic PCLs, only 4 eyes of the 450 (0.9%) demonstrated any signs of lenticular change, and these were only small localized white spots in the peripheral anterior cortex. None of the eyes in this six-year follow-up study developed any central cataractous changes. The endothelial cell loss in 405 eyes (90%) averaged 5 percent. A small group (10 eyes) had prolonged postoperative iritis, lasting six months, and also had an excessive cell loss, averaging 20 percent. In an early report of 43 second-generation posterior chamber lenses implanted since 1990,[15] these cases are also showing a cell loss of 5% or less. In this small initial series of collagen lenses, no cases of postoperative iritis were reported.

Since 1990, one United States investigator, Albert C. Neumann (Deland, Florida) has implanted four of the second-generation Fyodorov lenses. None of these lenses were apparently fixated by the zonule and all appeared to be slightly too short for true ciliary sulcus fixation, as they all subluxed slightly laterally. All of these eyes required topical steroids for a longer duration than is usually required for routine cataract-implant cases. One lens was finally removed for intractable iritis. This eye had two subsequent episodes of recurrent iritis. In Dr. Neumann's very limited series of phakic posterior chamber implantation, the average cell loss to-date is 11 percent.[16]

The second-generation Fyodorov lens has also been implanted in a few eyes by two surgeons in Turkey, Dr. Ertuk and Dr. Yilmaz. Dr. Yilmaz found, as did Dr. Neumann also, that the Fyodorov nomogram (see Table 7-3) seemed to produce overcorrections for myopia greater than -10.00.

Paul Fechner of Hanover-Gehrden, Germany, recently reported his initial experience with a German-manufactured Fyodorov IOL "clone" made of silicone (ADATOMED, GmbH, Munich).[17] He used superior limbal incisions 7.0 mm in length and selected the length of the IOL according to the formula "white-to-white-plus-0.5 mm." A peripheral iridectomy was made in each case and the incisions were sutured. Prednisone 250 mg was administered intravenously to help reduce the degree of iritis postoperatively. Dr. Fechner implanted 20 lenses in 18 patients with myopia from -8.00 to -23.00 between November 1992 and March 1993. As of September of 1993, he was encouraged with the early results and had not seen any vision loss due to cataract formation.

In the fall of 1993, clinical investigation of another Fyodorov lens "clone" was begun by STAAR Surgical (Bern, Switzerland). This lens is a collagen-silicone copolymer, similar to the Russian material, and has been implanted by Christian Skorpik in Austria, Vicenzo Assetto, Paolo Pesandro, and Stefano Benedetti in Italy, and recently by Roberto Zalvivar in Mendoza, Argentina.

The Future . . . Now?

The fact that approximately 3,000 IOLs have been implanted in the last eight years on four continents to correct refractive errors has established phakic intraocular lens implantation as a refractive surgical procedure whose "time has come." It has legitimately joined the ranks of the various keratorefractive procedures now also under development. The fates of currently used implant designs, materials, and methods will ultimately be determined by the long-term relationship between these intraocular prostheses and their surrounding contiguous structures.

We could say phakic implantation in the 1950s was in its infancy, the first-generation phakic IOLs of the 1980s moved the technology into its childhood, and the current generation of products in the early 1990s is at the adolescent stage of development. Does that mean that the fully grown art and science of the intraocular correction of the ametropias is imminent? There certainly seems to be no resistance on the part of the "visually handicapped" high ametropes.

The technical concepts associated with phakic implantation would certainly seem to be equally as appealing, not only to those who suffer the handicaps, but also to those whose hands may "heal" these handicapped. Its unique features already enumerated, not associated with keratorefractive approaches, include accuracy, immediacy, predictability, reversibility, stability, comfortability, familiarity, and frugality. But aside from all of these technical advantages to the healer and the "healee," perhaps the greatest effect of this adventurous endeavor is seen in the difference which this simple procedure makes in the quality of life for its beneficiaries. If our mission, as physicians, is to make a difference in our lifetime, this procedure—above all others—may have the potential to make one of the greatest differences. It may be summed up by the observation of Herb Kaufman after implanting the second eyes of his first five high myopes, "These are the happiest patients you've ever seen."[18]

Suggested Reading

Applegate RA, Howland HC: Magnification and visual acuity in refractive surgery. *Arch Ophthal*. Vol. III, Oct 1993; pp. 1335-1342.

Arciniegas A: Treatment of high myopia with a pars plana vitrectomy, posterior lensectomy, and scleral buckling in 360° (a modified Fukala). *J Oc Therapy & Surg*. Vol. 4, No. 1, Apr/May 1985; pp. 6-9.

Baikoff G: Phakic anterior chamber intraocular lenses. *Int. Ophthal. Clin*. Vol. 31, No. 1, 1991; pp. 75-86.

Baikoff G, Joly P: Comparison of minus power anterior chamber intraocular lenses and myopic epikeratoplasty in phakic eyes. *Refract Corneal Surg*. 1990; 6: 252-260.

Baikoff G: The refractive IOL in a phakic eye. *Ophthalmic Prac*. 1991; 9: 58-61, 80.

Barraquer J: Anterior chamber plastic lenses: results and conclusions from five years' experience. *Trans Ophthal Soc UK*. 79: 393-424, 1959.

Borley WE, Snyder AA: Surgical treatment of high myopia. *Trans Am Acad Ophthalmol Otolaryngol*. 1958; 62: 791-802.

Choyce DP: Baikoff-style anterior chamber lens used for high myopia in a phakic patient. *Oc Surg News*. Jan 15, 1992.

Choyce DP: Residual myopia after radial keratotomy successfully treated with Baikoff ZB5M IOLs. *Refract & Corneal Surg*. Vol. 9, Nov/Dec 1993; p. 475.

Colin J, Robinet A: Clear lensectomy and implantation of low-power posterior-chamber intraocular lens for the correction of high myopia. *Ophthalmology*. Vol. 101, No. 1, Jan. 1994; pp. 107-112.

Colin J, Mimouni F, Robinet A, et al: The surgical treatment of high myopia: comparison of epikeratoplasty, keratomileusis and minus power anterior chamber lenses. *Refract Corneal Surg*. 1990; 6: 245-251.

Curtin BJ, Whitmore MD: Long-term results of scleral reinforcement surgery. *Am J Ophthalmol*. 1987; 103: 544-548.

Curtin BJ: Scleral support of the posterior sclera, II: clinical results. *Am J Ophthalmol*. 1961; 52: 853-862.

Curtin BJ: Posterior staphyloma development in pathologic myopa. *Ann Ophthalmol*. 1982; 14: 655-658.

Curtin BJ: Surgical support of the posterior sclera, I: experimental results. *Am J Ophthalmol*. 1960; 49: 1341-1350.

Fechner PU, Worst JGF: A new concave intraocular lens for the correction of myopia. *Eur J Implant Ref Surg*. Vol. 1, Mar 1989; pp. 41-43.

Fechner PU, Strobal J, Wichmann W: Correction of myopia by implantation of a concave Worst iris-claw lens into phakic eyes. *Refract & Corneal Surg*. Vol. 7, Jul/Aug 1991; pp. 286-298.

Fechner PU, van der Heijde GL, Worst JGF: The correction of myopia by lens implantation into phakic eyes. *Am J Ophthalmol*. 107: 659, 1989.

Fechner PU, van der Heijde GL, Worst JGF: The correction of myopia by lens implantation into phakic eyes (correspondence). *Am J Ophthalmol*. 108: 465, 1989.

Fyodorov SN: Two cases of correction of pronounced unilateral myopia with the use of an anterior chamber lens. *Vestn Optalmol*. 82(3): 27-38, 1969.

Fyodorov SN, Zuyek VK, Tumanyan ER, Larionov YeV: Analysis of long-term clinical and functional results of intraocular correction of high myopia. *Ophthalmosurgery*. 1990; 2: 3-6.

Goldberg MF: Clear lens extraction for axial myopia. *Ophthalmology*. 94: 571-582, 1987.

Hanczye P: Surgical treatment of progressive high myopia. *Klin Oczna*. 1973; 43: 803-811.

Holladay JT: Refractive power calculations for intraocular lenses in the phakic eye. *AJO*. 116: 63-66, Jul 1993.

Jacob-LaBarre JT, Assouline M, Conway MD, Thompson HW, McDonald M: Effects of scleral reinforcement on the elongation of growing cat eyes. *Arch Ophthal*. Vol III, Jul 1993; pp. 979-986.

Jacob-LaBarre JT, Assouline M, Hart L, McDonald M: Polymeric bands for scleral reinforcement surgery: biocompatibility and clincal results for 15 different materials. Read before the Fourth World Biomaterials Congress; April 24-28, 1992; Berlin, Germany.

Koch PS: Hyperic lensectomy study under way in U.S., by Jim Knaub for *Oc Surg News*. Vol. 11, No. 15, Aug 1, 1993.

Miller WW: Surgical treatment of degenerative myopia: scleral reinforment. *Trans Am Acad Ophthalmol Otalyngol*. 1974; 78: OP896-OP910.

Mimouni F, Colin J, Koffi V, Bonnet P: Damage to the corneal endothelium from anterior chamber intraocular lenses in phakic myopic eyes. *Refract Corneal Surg.* 7: 277, 1991.

Nesterov AP, Svirin AV, Antipova OA: Scleral reinforcement. *J Ocul Therapy Surg.* 1984; 3: 255-261.

Perez-Santonja JJ, Bueno JL, Meza J, Garcia-Sandoval B, Serrano JM, Zato MA: Ischemic optic neuropathy after intraocular lens implantation to correct high myopia in a phakic patient. *J Cat Refract Surg.* Vol. 19, Sept 1993; pp. 651-654.

Porter D, Peiffer R, Eifrig E, Boyd J: Experimental evaluation of a phakic anterior chamber implant in a primate model, Part II: Pathology. *J Cat Refract Surg.* 17:342, 1991.

Praeger DL: Innovations and creativity in contemporary opthalmology: preliminary experience with the phakic myopic intraocular lens. *Ann Ophthal.* 20: 456-462, 1988.

Praeger DL: Phakic myopic intraocular lenses—an alternative to kerato- lenticulorefractive procedures. *Ann Ophthal.* Jul 1988; p. 246.

Rijneveld WJ, Beekhuis WH, Hassman EF, Dellgert M, Geerards A: Iris claw lens: anterior and posterior iris surface fixation in the absense of capsular support during penetrating keratoplasty. *Refract & Corneal Surg.* 10: 14-19, 1994.

Saragoussi JJ, Othenin-Girard P, Pouliquen YJM: Ocular damage after implantation of over-sized minus power anterior chamber intraocular lenses in myopic phakic eyes: case reports. *Refract & Corneal Surg.* Vol. 9, Mar/Apr 1993; pp. 105-109.

Thompson FB: Scleral reinforcement for severe myopia: case report demonstrating long-term viability of scleral implant. *Ann Ophthalmol.* 1982; 14: 94-95.

Thompson FB: A simplified scleral reinforcement technique. *Am J Ophthalmol.* 1978; 86: 782-790.

Thompson FB: Scleral reinforcement for high myopia. *Ophthalmic Surg.* 1985; 16: 90-94.

Thompson FB, Turner AF: Computed axial tomography on highly myopic eyes following scleral reinforcement surgery. *Ophthalmic Surg.* 1992; 23: 253-259.

van der Heijde GL: Some optical aspects of implantation of an IOL in a myopic eye. *Eur J Implant Ref Surg.* Vol. 1, Dec 1989; pp. 245-248.

Verzella F: Lensectomy. *Ophthal Forum.* Vol. 3, No. 3, 1985; p. 191.

Verzella F: High myopia: in-the-bag refractive implantation. *Ophthal Forum.* Vol. 3, No. 3, 1985; pp. 174-175.

Verzella F: High myopia: low-power intraocular lens in the posterior chamber for optical purposes. *J Kerato-Refract Soc.* May/Jun 1985; pp. 20-22.

Waring GO III: Phakic intraocular lenses for the correction of myopia. Where do we go from here? *Refract Corneal Surg.* 7: 275, 1991.

Werblin TP: Should we consider clear lens extraction for routine refractive surgery. *Refract & Corneal Surg.* Vol. 8, Nov/Dec 1992; pp. 480-481.

Whitmore WG, Curtin BJ: Scleral reinforcement: two case reports. *Ophthalmic Surg.* 1987; 18: 503-505.

Whitmore WG, Harrison W, Curtin BJ: Scleral reinforcement in rabbits using synthetic graft materials. *Ophthalmic Surg.* 1990; 21: 327-330.

Wilson SE: The correction of myopia with phakic intraocular lenses. *AJO.* Vol. 115, No. 2, Feb 1993; pp. 249-251.

Wilson SE: The correction of myopia by lens implantation into phakic eyes (correspondence). *Am J Ophthalmol.* 108:465, 1989.

References

1. Sanders DR: personal communication.

2. Holladay JT: Refractive power calculations for intraocular lenses in the phakic eye. *AJO* 116: 63-66, July 1993.

3. Saragoussi JJ, Othenin-Girard P, Poullquen Y: Ocular damage after implantation of oversized minus power anterior chamber intraocular lenses in myopic phakic eyes: case reports. *Ref. & Corn. Surg.* 9:105- 109, Mar-Apr 1993.

4. Mimourri F, Colin J, Koffè V, Bonnet P: Damage to the corneal endothelium from anterior chamber intraocular lenses in phakic myopic eyes. *Ref. & Corn. Surg.* 7:277-281, Jul-Aug 1991.

5. Saragoussi JJ, Cotinat J, Renard G, Savoldelli M, Abenhaim A, Pouliquen Y: Damage to the corneal endothelium by minus power anterior chamber intraocular lenses. *Ref. & Corn. Surg.* 7:282-285, Jul- Aug 1991.

6. Baikoff G: Les implants myopiques, personal written communication, Nov 1993.

7. Kaufman HE: Letter to the editor: phakic ACLs. *Oc. Surg. News* Jun 15, 1992.

8. Alió JL, Ruiz-Moreno JM, Artola A: Retinal detachment as a potential hazard in surgical correction of severe myopia with phakic anterior chamber lenses. *AJO.* 115:143-148, Feb 1993.

9. Praeger DL, Momose A, Muroff LL: Thirty-six month follow-up of a contemporary phakic intraocular lens for the surgical correction of myopia. *Ann Ophthal.* 23:6-10, 1991.

10. Fechner PU, Wichmann W: Correction of myopia by implantation of minus optic (Worst iris-claw) lenses into the anterior chamber of phakic eyes. *Europ. J Impl. Ref. Surg.* 5:55-59, Mar 1993.

11. Menezo JL: Time-tested iris-claw design works well in phakic myopes. *Oc. Surg. New.* Apr 1993.

12. Alió Y Sanz JL: Interview. *Oc. Surg. News.* June 15, 1993, p.1, and letter to the editor. *Oc. Surg. News.* Jan 1, 1994, p. 7.

13. Worst JGF: Letter to the editor. *Oc. Surg. News.* Jan 1, 1994, p. 7.

14. Fyodorov SN, Zuyev VK, Tumanyan NR, Suheil AJ: Clinical and functional follow-up of minus IOL implantation in high-grade myopia. *Ophthalmosurgery.* 2:12-17, 1993.

15. Fyodorov SN, Zuyev VK, Aznabayev BM: Intraocular correction of high myopia with negative posterior chamber lens. *Ophthalmosurgery.* 3:57-58, 1991.

16. Neumann AC: presented at the ESCRS Annual Symposium, Innsbruck, Austria, September 1993, by Schonfeld AR: Update on three IOLs for myopia. *Oc. Surg. News.* Dec 1, 1993.

17. Fechner PU: presented at the ESCRS Annual Symposium, Innsbruck, Austria, September 1993, by Schonfeld AR: Phakic PCL is promising for high myopia. *Oc. Surg. News. Int'l. Ed.* 4:12, Dec 1993.

18. Kaufman HE: Phakic IOL study results are promising. *Oc. Surg. News.* Jun 15, 1993.

Appendix I

Surgical Nomograms

Kershner Nomograms

Kershner Arcuate Keratotomy
System Nomograms

Correction (Diopters)	Optical Zone (mm)	Arcuate Incision Length (mm)
<1.0	10	2.5 (1)
1.0	9	2.5 (1)
1.5	9	3.0 (1)
2.0	8	2.5 (2)
2.5	9 / 7	2.5 (2)
3.0	9 / 7	3.0 (2)
3.5	8 / 7	3.0 (2)
4.0	6	2.0 (2)
4.5	6	2.5 (2)
5.0	6	3.0 (2)
5.5	5	2.0 (2)
6.0	5	2.5 (2)

Corrected for age 60 +. Arcs placed on steepest axis of astigmatism (plus cylinder). Pachymetry at incision site, square diamond keratome set to 100% of pachymetry. Mark arcuate incisions and optical zone with Kershner One-Step Marker. Cataract keratotomy at 10 mm, 9 mm, or 8 mm only.

Kershner Surgical Worksheet

**Orange Grove Center
for Corrective Eye Surgery**
Robert M. Kershner, M.D., P.C., F.A.C.S.
1925 W. Orange Grove Road • Suite 303
Tucson, AZ 85704-1117
(602) 797-2020

Patient Name: _____
Age: _____ Occupation: _____
Dominent Eye: _____ Date: _____

V R20/___   V R20/___   J R____
sc L20/___   cc L20/___   L____

C R   .   +   .   X _____

___ L   .   +   .   X _____

K R   .   V   .   H ___°

___ L   .   V   .   H ___°

WEARS: R _____ . ___ + ___ . ___ X _____
Glasses L _____ . ___ + ___ . ___ X _____
ADD: _____ Last Rx _____

WEARS: R _____
Contacts L _____
Last Rx: _____

O.D.

O.S.

O.Z. ___ . ___ mm   ARC LENGTH ___ . ___ mm

O.Z. ___ . ___ mm   ARC LENGTH ___ . ___ mm

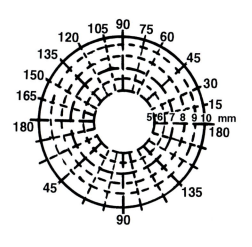

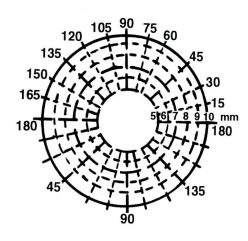

PACHYMETRY _____

PACHYMETRY _____

Kershner Nomogram

When the surgeon elects to perform keratolenticuloplasty, certain rules should be kept in mind. I call these the caveats of KLP.

1. Always slightly undercorrect the pre-existing astigmatism. You can always do more surgery later if needed, but it may be difficult to undo what you have already done if you have done too much. Remember, in older patients, the less elastic cornea responds with greater changes in curvature for a given amount of surgery.

2. It is best to avoid arcuate incisions inside the 7-mm optical zone, unless needed. That is, if it is possible to achieve the same degree of correction at 7 mm with a slightly larger arc, this is to be preferred over a smaller arc at a 6-mm or 5-mm optical zone. In other words, larger incisions are always preferred further away from the optical zone even though their effect decreases as the distance from the optical zone increases.

3. Arcuate incisions should never exceed 60° in length at any optical zone and, ideally, the largest arc should be no greater than 45° or 3 mm.

4. 85% to 95% depth is ideal for an astigmatic effect. Avoid perforating the cornea needlessly, it makes phacoemulsification and maintaining the anterior chamber more difficult.

5. Whenever possible, if a single arcuate incision will suffice, it will be preferable than using two smaller incisions.

6. Always attempt to keep the arcuate incision closest to the surgeon for the keratotomy into the anterior chamber. Place this incision anterior to the limbal vascular arcade at 10 mm, 9 mm or 8 mm. Avoid using the arcuate incision for the subsequent cataract surgery if it is closer to the optical center of the eye than the 8-mm optical zone.

7. To avoid full thickness penetration, avoid pressing on the globe with another instrument during the creation of the arcuate incision. Holding the eye, if required at all, is best performed with a toothed forceps at the conjunctiva. Keep the keratome fully applanated with both footplates and avoid tilting the handle.

8. It is easier to visualize the marks and incise the cornea if the cornea is kept slightly dry.

9. Avoid using marking inks. They obscure visualization for subsequent procedures of cataract surgery. A clean marker gently pressed onto the epithelium will create a visible mark that will be more than satisfactory as a guideline to creating the incision.

10. Simply placing your arcuate corneal cataract incision on the axis of steepest astigmatism will almost always improve the refractive result. However, operating on the incorrect axis will always make the refractive result worse. Axis is crucial. Never operate greater than 15° off axis.

Thornton Nomograms

Incision Lengths at
Varying Optical Zones

Length	5 mm OZ	6 mm OZ	7 mm OZ	8 mm OZ
20°	0.9 mm	1.0 mm	1.2 mm	1.4 mm
25°	1.0 mm	1.3 mm	1.5 mm	1.7 mm
30°	1.3 mm	1.5 mm	1.8 mm	2.0 mm
35°	1.5 mm	1.8 mm	2.1 mm	2.4 mm
40°	1.7 mm	2.0 mm	2.4 mm	2.7 mm
45°	1.9 mm	2.3 mm	2.7 mm	3.1 mm
50°	2.1 mm	2.5 mm	2.9 mm	3.4 mm

Thornton Nomogram for Astigmatic Keratotomy

Assumes cuts 98% deep (almost to Descemet's membrane) along the full length of the incision.
The Sum of the Modifiers = The Theoretical Target Cylinder

Age: For every year below age 30, add $1/2$% to the astigmatic error. For every year above age 30, subtract $1/2$% per year.

Sex: In premenopausal women (under age 40) subtract three years from actual age.

IOP: For every mm IOP below 12, add 2% to cylinder error. For every mm IOP above 15, subtract 2% from amount of cylinder.

Cylinder Corrected by Paired Arcuate Transverse Incisions

Chord Length of One Pair
Arcuate Transverse Incisions

Theoretical Cylinder	Degrees Arc
0.50 D	20°
0.75 D	23°
1.00 D	25°
1.25 D	28°
1.50 D	32°
1.75 D	35°
2.00 D	38°
2.25 D	42°
2.50 D	45°

One pair always placed at the 7 mm OZ

Chord Length of Two Pair
Arcuate Transverse Incisions

Theoretical Cylinder	Degrees Arc
2.00 D	23°
2.25 D	27°
2.50 D	31°
2.75 D	35°
3.00 D	39°
3.25 D	43°
3.50 D	47°
3.75 D	48°

Two pairs outer at the 8
inner at the 6

Chord Length of Three Pair
Arcuate Transverse Incisions

Theoretical Cylinder	Degrees Arc
3.25 D	22°
3.50 D	26°
3.75 D	30°
4.00 D	35°
4.25 D	40°
4.50 D	45°
4.75 D	50°
5.00 D	54°

Three pairs
outer just outside the 8
middle incision at the 7
inner just inside the 6

Smaller OZ (5.5 mm to 7.5 mm) → 0.50 D to 1.00 D more

Durrie/Schumer Nomograms

Durrie/Schumer Nomogram

ASTIGMATISM REDUCTION CLINICAL TRIAL

EXPLANATION FOR USE OF NOMOGRAM

- Identify patient's age and the diopters of refractive cylinder that you wish to correct.

- Find the patient's age in the first column on the left.

- Move to the right until you've reached the surgery result closest to the refractive cylinder of the patient. In order to avoid overcorrection, it is suggested that you select a surgical goal somewhat less than the actual refractive cylinder. The column heading tells you which surgery is needed to achieve this result.

EXAMPLE

45-year-old patient with a refractive cylinder of 3.75

- 3.75 falls between 2.60 and 3.90

- A single 90° ARC-T or a paired 45° ARC-T will correct 2.60 diopters of cylinder

- A paired 60° ARC-T will correct 3.90 diopters of cylinder

- The recommendation in this case is to do a paired 45° or a single 90° ARC-T

EXPECTED SURGICAL RESULTS WERE CALCULATED
USING LINDSTROM'S FORMULA

$$\Delta D = [100 + (AGE - 30) \times 2] \times [\Delta D \text{ at age } 30] \times 0.01$$

The arcuate keratotomy nomogram.

Durrie/Schumer Nomogram

AGE	Surgical option				
	2 X 30°		2 X 45°		
	1 X 45°	1 X 60°	1 X 90°	2 X 60°	2 X 90°
20	0.80	1.20	1.60	2.40	3.20
21	0.82	1.23	1.64	2.46	3.28
22	0.84	1.26	1.68	2.52	3.36
23	0.86	1.29	1.72	2.58	3.44
24	0.88	1.32	1.76	2.64	3.52
25	0.90	1.35	1.80	2.70	3.60
26	0.92	1.38	1.84	2.76	3.68
27	0.94	1.41	1.88	2.82	3.76
28	0.96	1.44	1.92	2.88	3.84
29	0.98	1.47	1.96	2.94	3.92
30	1.00	1.50	2.00	3.00	4.00
31	1.02	1.53	2.04	3.06	4.08
32	1.04	1.56	2.08	3.12	4.16
33	1.06	1.59	2.12	3.18	4.24
34	1.08	1.62	2.16	3.24	4.32
35	1.10	1.65	2.20	3.30	4.40
36	1.12	1.68	2.24	3.36	4.48
37	1.14	1.71	2.28	3.42	4.56
38	1.16	1.74	2.32	3.48	4.64
39	1.18	1.77	2.36	3.54	4.72
40	1.20	1.80	2.40	3.60	4.80
41	1.22	1.83	2.44	3.66	4.88
42	1.24	1.86	2.48	3.72	4.96
43	1.26	1.89	2.52	3.78	5.04
44	1.28	1.92	2.56	3.84	5.12
45	1.30	1.95	2.60	3.90	5.20
46	1.32	1.98	2.64	3.96	5.28
47	1.34	2.01	2.68	4.02	5.36
48	1.36	2.04	2.72	4.08	5.44
49	1.38	2.07	2.76	4.14	5.52
50	1.40	2.10	2.80	4.20	5.60
51	1.42	2.13	2.84	4.26	5.68
52	1.44	2.16	2.88	4.32	5.76
53	1.46	2.19	2.92	4.38	5.84
54	1.48	2.22	2.96	4.44	5.92
55	1.50	2.25	3.00	4.50	6.00
56	1.52	2.28	3.04	4.56	6.08
57	1.54	2.31	3.08	4.62	6.16
58	1.56	2.34	3.12	4.68	6.24
59	1.58	2.37	3.16	4.74	6.32
60	1.60	2.40	3.20	4.80	6.40
61	1.62	2.43	3.24	4.86	6.48
62	1.64	2.46	3.28	4.92	6.56
63	1.66	2.49	3.32	4.98	6.64
64	1.68	2.52	3.36	5.04	6.72
65	1.70	2.55	3.40	5.10	6.80
66	1.72	2.58	3.44	5.16	6.88
67	1.74	2.61	3.48	5.22	6.96
68	1.76	2.64	3.52	5.28	7.04
69	1.78	2.67	3.56	5.34	7.12
70	1.80	2.70	3.60	5.40	7.20
71	1.82	2.73	3.64	5.46	7.28
72	1.84	2.76	3.68	5.52	7.36
73	1.86	2.79	3.72	5.58	7.44
74	1.88	2.82	3.76	5.64	7.52
75	1.90	2.85	3.80	5.70	7.60
AGE	1 X 45°	1 X 60°	1 X 90°	2 X 60°	2 X 90°
	2 X 30°		2 X 45°		

The arcuate keratotomy nomogram continued.

Durrie/Schumer Nomogram

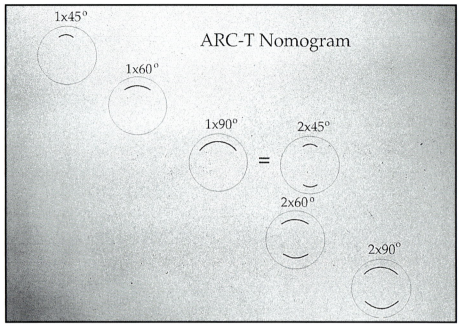

The arcuate keratotomy nomogram continued.

Durrie/Schumer Worksheet

TRK OPERATIVE PLAN

NAME_____ AGE _____ SEX_____

DATE OF SURGERY_____ DOMINANT EYE_____ DATE OF LAST VISIT_____

OD

	Today	Last Visit	Original
VASC			
VACC			

MRx Today _____ _____ x _____
    Last visit _____ _____ x _____
    Original _____ _____ x _____

CRx Today _____ _____ x _____
    Last visit _____ _____ x _____
    Original _____ _____ x _____

SE   Today _____
    Last visit _____
    Original _____

K   Today _____x_____ _____x_____
    Last vist _____x_____ _____x_____
    Original _____x_____ _____x_____

Pachymetry

C_____
M_____
I_____
L_____
S_____

DEPTH _____

RED = PLANNED PROCEDURE
BLUE = PREVIOUS INCISIONS

OS

	Today	Last Visit	Original
VASC			
VACC			

MRx Today _____ _____ x _____
    Last visit _____ _____ x _____
    Original _____ _____ x _____

CRx Today _____ _____ x _____
    Last visit _____ _____ x _____
    Original _____ _____ x _____

SE   Today _____
    Last visit _____
    Original _____

K   Today _____x_____ _____x_____
    Last vist _____x_____ _____x_____
    Original _____x_____ _____x_____

Pachymetry

C_____
M_____
I_____
L_____
S_____

DEPTH _____

PHYSICIAN'S SIGNATURE

Refractive surgery worksheet.

Appendix II

Suggested Readings

Cohen KL, Tripoli NK, Noecher RJ: Prospective analysis of photokeratoscopy for arcuate keratotomy to reduce postkeratoplasty astigmatism. *Refract Corneal Surg.* 1989, Nov-Dec;5(6):388-93.

Davison JA: Transverse astigmatic keratotomy combined with phacoemulsification and intraocular lens implantation. *J Cataract Refract Surg.* 1989, Jan;15(1):32-7.

Duffey RJ, Jain VN, Tchah H, Hofmann RF, Lindstrom RL: Paired arcuate keratotomy: a surgical approach to mixed and myopic astigmatism. *Arch Ophthalmol.* 1988, Aug;106(8):1130-5.

Duffy RJ, Vivanti NJ, et al: Paired arcuate keratotomy: a surgical approach to mixed and myopic astigmatism. *Arch Ophthal.* 1988, 103;477-488.

Frangieh GT, Kwitko S, McDonnell PJ: Prospective corneal topogaphic analysis in surgery for postkeratoplasty astigmatism. *Arch Ophthalmol.* 1991, Apr;109(4):506-10.

Grene RB, Lindstrom RL: Astigmatic keratotomy in the refractive patient: the ARC-T study: in Gills JP, Thornton SP, Martin RG, Sanders DR, eds, *Surgical Treatment of Astigmatism.* Thorofare, NJ, SLACK, Inc., 1994.

Grene RB: Astigmatism Chapter. In: Roy FH, ed, *Ophthalmic Surgery: Approaches of the Masters.* Philadelphia, PA, Lee & Febiger, In press.

Grene RB, Kenyon KR, Durrie DS, Lindstrom RL, Price FW, Whitson WE, Bodner BI, Binder PS, Gelender H: Astigmatism Reduction Clinical Trial: a multi-center prospective evaluation of the surgical results of arcuate keratotomy for the reduction of astigmatism, 1993. Submitted.

Hall GW, Campion M, Sorenson CM, Monthofer S: Reduction of corneal astigmatism at cataract surgery. *J Cataract Refract Surg.* 1991, July;17(4):407-14.

Hanna KD, Jouve PE, Waring GO 3d, Ciarlet PG: Computer simulation of arcuate keratotomy for astigmatism. *Refract Corneal Surg.* 1992, Mar-Apr;8(2):152-63.

Hofmann RF: The surgical correction of idiopathic astigmatism. *Refractive Corneal Surgery.* Thorofare, NJ, SLACK, Inc., pp 241-290, 1986.

Holladay JT, Cravy TV, Koch DD: Calculating the surgically induced refractive change following ocular surgery. *J Cataract Refract Surg.* 1992, 18:429-443.

Ibrahim O, Hussein HA, el-Sahn MF, el-Nawawy S, Kassem A, Waring GO 3d: Trapesoidal keratotomy for the correction of naturally occurring astigmatism. *Arch Ophthalmol.* 1991, Oct;109(10):1374-81.

Jaffe NS, Clayman HM: The pathophysicology of corneal astigmatism after cataract extraction. *Trans Am Acad Ophthalmol Otolaryngol.* 79 Jul/Aug OP-628-OP-630, 1975.

Jaffe NS, Clayman HM: The pathophysicology of corneal astigmatism after cataract extraction. *Trans Am Acad Ophthalmol Otolaryngol.* 79 Jul/Aug OP-616, 1975.

Koch DD, Lindstrom RL: Controlling astigmatism in cataract surgery. Seminars in Ophthalmology. Dec 1992;Vol 7-4:224-233.

Krumeich JH, Knuelle A: Circular keratotomy for the correction of astigmatism. *Refract Corneal Surg.* 1992, May-Jun;8(3):204-10.

Lebuisson DA: Transverse incisions in the treatment of astigmatism combined with radial keratotomy. Preliminary results. *Dev Ophthalmol.* 1989, 18:185-91.

Lindstrom RL: Surgical correction of postoperative astigmatism. *Indian J. Ophthalmol.* 1990, July-Sep;38(3):114-23.

Lindstrom RL, Lindquist TD: Surgical correction of postoperative astigmatism. *Cornea.* 1988; 7(2):138-48.

Lindstrom RL: Lans distinguished refractive surgery lecture: the surgical correction of astigmatism; a clinician's perspective. *Refractive & Corneal Surgery.* Nov/Dec 1990; Vol 6:441-454.

Lipshitz I, Mayron Y, Loewenstein A: Combined transverse and interrupted radial keratotomy for compound myopic astigmatism. *Refract Corneal Surg.* 1992, Jul-Aug;8(4):280-5.

Lundergun MK, Rowsey JJ: Relaxing incisions: corneal topography. *Ophthalmology.* 1985, 92:1226-1236.

McCluskey DJ, Villasenor R, McDonnell PJ: Prospective topographic analysis in peripheral arcuate keratotomy for astigmatism. *Ophthalmic Surg.* 1990, July;21(7):464-71.

Maguire LJ, Bourne WM: Corneal topography of transverse keratotomies for astigmatism after penetrating keratoplasty. *AM J Ophthalmol.* 1989, Apr15;107(4):323-30.

Maloney WF: Transverse astigmatic keratotomy: an integral part of small incision cataract surgery. *J Cataract Refract Surg.* 1992, Mar;18:190-194.

Merlin U: Curved keratotomy procedure for congenital astigmatism. *J Refract Surg.* 1987, 3:92-97.

Neumann AC, McCarty GR, Sanders DR, Raanan MG: Refractive evaluation of astigmatic keratotomy procedures. *J Cataract Refract Surg.* 1989, Jan;15(1):25-31.

Nordan LT, Grene RB: The importance of corneal aspericity and irregular astigmatism in refractive surgery. *Refract Corneal Surg.* 1990, May-June;6(3):200-4.

Nordan LT, Maxwell WA, Davison JA: *The Surgical Rehabilitation of Vision.* Gower Medical Publishing, 1992, 23-28.

Osher RH: Paired transverse relaxing keratotomy: a combined technique for reducing astigmatism. *J Cataract Refract Surg.* 1989, Jan;15(1):32-7.

Park K, Lee JH: Surgical correction of astigmatism using paired T-incisions. *Korean J. Ophthalmol.* 1989, Dec;3(2):61-4.

Price WP, Grene RB, Marks RC: Astigmatism Reduction Clinial Trial: one month & six month data with analysis of the results of two-stage astigmatic/myopic surgery versus one-stage surgery. Submitted.

Price WP, Grene RB, Marks RC: Astigmatism Reduction Clinial Trial: a multi-center evaluation of the predicability of arcuate keratotomy. Evaluation of surgical nomogram predictability. Submitted.

Saragoussi JJ, Abenhaim A, Pouliquen Y: Results of transverse incisions in surgical correction of severe post-keratoplasty astigmatism. *J Fr Ophthalmol.* 1990, 13(10):492-9.

Saragoussi JJ, Abenhaim A, Waked N, Koster HR, Pouliquan YJ: Results of transverse keratotomies for astigmatism after penetrating keratoplasty: a retrospective study of 48 consecutive cases. *Refract Corneal Surg.* 1992, Jan-Feb; 8(1):33-8.

Schneider DM, Draghic T, Murthy RK: Combined myopia and astigmatism surgery: review of 350 cases. *J Cataract Refract Surg.* 1992, Jul;18(4):370-4.

Thornton SP: Transverse astigmatic keratotomy. *J Cataract Refract Surg.* 1991, Nov;17(6):861.

Thornton SP, Sanders DR: Graded nonintersecting transverse incisions for correction of idiopathic astigmatism. *J Cataract Refract Surg.* 1987, Jan;13(1):27-31.

Index